The DASH Diet Solution and 60 Day Weight Loss and Fitness Journal

The Dash Diet Solution
and 60 Day Weight Loss and Fitness Journal

ISBN: 978-1-936583-29-4

Note: This book is not intended to provide medical advice or take the place of your doctor's advice. It is always important to consult your physician before beginning any diet or exercise program. The DASH Diet has been researched, and endorsed by the National Institute of Health but neither the publisher nor editor take responsibility for any possible consequences from its use and nothing in this book is intended as a substitute for medical advice. Additionally, it is always good to consult your physican before beginning any exercise and diet program..

Learning Visions
1710 Moorpark Road Suite #213
Thousand Oaks, Ca 91362
For other books from Learning Visions or
from its imprint, Lakewood Publishing, see:
www.lakewoodpublishing.com

The DASH Diet Solution and 60 Day Weight Loss and Fitness Journal

Learning Visions

Acknowledgement
DASH Diet and other nutrition, heatlh and fitness information provided courtesy of The National Institute of Health, The National Heart, Lung and Blood Institute of the NIH and by the CDC (Center for Disease Control)

Table of Contents

God, grant me the Serenity
to accept the things I cannot change,
the courage to change the things I can,
and the wisdom to know the difference.

--Opening lines of the "Serenity Prayer"
by Reinhold Niebuhr

1

"The #1 Diet in America"

In 2012, a panel of 22 diet and nutrition experts evaluated 25 diets for *U.S. News and World Report*. From a list that included the *Atkins Diet* and the *South Beach Diet*, as well as some of the most popular commercially packaged diets, these experts chose the *DASH Diet* as the "#1 Best Overall Diet". In addition to promoting weight loss, they chose DASH for three reasons: (1) DASH is based on good nutrition, (2) it includes low amounts of daily salt (sodium), and (3) it is easy to follow without relying on processed foods. In addition to being the "Best Overall Diet", *U.S. News and World Report* also chose DASH as the best diet for healthy eating and as a top recommended diet for diabetics. DASH was praised for being a diet that people could easily follow for a lifetime.

DASH was unique among the diets that *U.S. New and World Report* evaluated because began as a U.S. government study of blood pressure. This book shares the recommendations from that research, and shows you how to easily incorporate the DASH principles into your daily ife.

Every year, new fad diets appear that promise fast results but only deliver short term benefits, if they deliver any benefits at all. Not only are these quick-fix diets often unhealthy, but because they don't result in lifestyle changes, any weight that is lost can be all too quickly regained.

DASH is that rare diet that promotes weight loss at the same time it develops healthy habits that will be easy to continue even after your weight loss goals have been met.

DASH does not use food gimmicks, and you don't have to starve yourself to lose weight. DASH promotes good health along with weight loss. It will help you make good food choices using a few simple principles that are easy to remember and follow wherever you are. Best of all, after you have achieved your desired weight with DASH, you will have accomplished more than losing pounds. You will have also learned how easy it is to change the way you think about food, you will understand the importance of recognizing the sodium and fat in your diet and how they affect your weight and health, and you will have learned how to lose weight—and how to keep the excess pounds off.

What the Experts Are Saying

DASH, which is an acronym for "Dietary Approaches to Stop Hypertension", has been shown in National Institute of Health studies to promote weight loss at the same time it improves overall health. In a major study of 412 participants, the National Heart, Lung and Blood Institute (NHLBI) found that, in addition to promoting weight loss, the DASH Diet lowered cholesterol, reduced or eliminated hypertension, reduced the risk of diabetes, and—perhaps most important of all—was effective in fighting two of the leading causes of death in the United States: heart attacks and strokes.

All that, and weight loss, too. It's no wonder that *U.S. News and World Report* was impressed.

DASH began as an NHLBI study of blood pressure. The first research participants were adults with systolic blood pressures of less than 160 mmHg and diastolic pressures of 80–95 mmHg (160/80-95). The researchers divided them into three groups, and gave each group a different eating plan. One plan had foods similar to what many Americans regularly eat. The second plan also had foods that many Americans regularly eat, but it added more fruits and vegetables. The third plan was the DASH diet. All three plans included about 3,000 milligrams of sodium daily, a fairly typical amount of sodium for many Americans.

None of the plans were vegetarian or used specialty foods, but the results were dramatic. Participants who followed the plan that included more fruits and vegetables or who used the DASH eating plan significantly reduced blood pressure. But those who were on the DASH eating plan had the greatest change, especially for participants with high blood pressure. And the improvement happened quickly—within two weeks of starting the plan.

The second DASH study had participants randomly divided into groups that would follow either a typical American diet or DASH. They were grouped into three different sodium (salt) levels and followed for a month.

The group with the highest level of sodium consumed about 3,300 milligrams of sodium per day, typical of the average American diet. Another group was given the lowest amount of sodium, about 1,500 milligrams per day. The third group had an intermediate amount—2,300 milligrams per day.

Results showed that reducing sodium lowered blood pressure for both of the lower groups. At each sodium level, blood pressure was lower on the DASH eating plan than on the other eating plan. The group that combined the DASH eating plan with the lowest sodium level (1500 milligrams per day) experienced the most dramatic results. Not surprisingly, participants with high blood pressure showed the greatest reductions, but even people with prehypertension also had large decreases. Even participants who did not follow DASH completely showed significant improvement in blood pressure—and they also showed another benefit as well: weight loss.

While Americans tend to worry about their weight, they often forget that high blood pressure and excess weight frequently go hand-in-hand. Weight gain is easy to observe, but high blood pressure is often called "the silent killer" because it can be asymptomatic. Maintaining a healthy weight and blood pressure through good eating habits does not only mean looking your best—it also can add years to your life.

How Do I Begin the DASH?

The DASH eating plan is easy to remember and easy to follow. It uses no specially prepared foods or dietary gimmicks. You just need to identify how many calories you need every day (see Chapter 4) and then match that number with the recommended daily servings of various food groups. *The DASH Diet Solution* lists diet plans for several calorie levels and Chapter 8 shows you how easy they are to use. The *60 Day Weight Loss and Fitness Journal* that begins on page 135 includes a daily checklist that makes DASH even easier to follow.

With its emphasis on lean protein, vegetables, fruit and fiber, DASH also helps you avoid the blood sugar fluctuations that often lead to broken diets. In fact, the *U.S. News and World Report* panel also chose DASH as the "Best Diabetes Diet" because it can help prevent Type 2 diabetes (a disease that is very diet-related) and because it helps people who already have diabetes to better manage the disease. (Of course, it is important for everyone to consult a doctor before beginning any diet—and even more important if you have an illness or chronic disease.)

The DASH Diet Solution is an easy-to-follow diet that reduces the risks of high blood pressure, and will help you develop eating habits to lose weight and keep it off, and will help fight or prevent many common diseases.

The DASH Eating Plan

The DASH Diet centers around fruits, vegetables, fat-free or low-fat dairy products, lean meats and whole grains. It minimizes the role of processed and packaged foods and reduces the sugar, fats, cholesterol and additives—including salt—that are so much a part of the modern diet. One in three Americans have high blood pressure and often don't know it. In addition to reducing the negative impact of too much salt in your diet, the DASH Diet also increases the good nutrients that are associated with lowering blood pressure—mainly potassium, magnesium, calcium, protein and fiber.

The DASH Diet Solution and 60 Day Weight less and Fitness Journal is a practical and interactive diet guide. In the next chapters, you will learn your BMI, how many calories you need based on your personal daily activity level, how to measure your target heart rate, and how to choose the right DASH plan for you. There are DASH plans at four different calorie levels, a week of sample menus, recipes, exercise tips, and a variety of interactive activities and questionnaires throughout the book all designed to help you succeed on DASH. When you are ready, you can begin the DASH Diet, with the help of the most essential part of this book—your personal DASH Diet journal.

How Keeping a Diet Journal Helps

Keeping a written record of your daily diet and exercise is important if you want to succeed in the difficult task of changing habits and losing weight. The *DASH Solution* journal, which begins on page 135, lets you track your progress

Using your journal, you will check off the daily DASH food group servings, make note of your food choices and record your daily exercise. Writing in your journal will keep you on track during times when you are most likely to make poor dietary choices, for example, when under stress, experiencing difficult life changes, at holidays, or even on vacation when daily routines can be so difficult to follow. Certain places and even people can also trigger dieting problems. Your diet journal will help you identify and plan for these problem situations in advance.

If You Aren't Ready to Diet Yet, a Journal Can Help

If you finish reading The DASH Diet Solution, but you are not ready to diet yet, you can still use your journal to help get motivated. Even if you are not dieting, writing in the journal every day will make you more aware of your current habits and what you need to do when you are ready to make changes.

Even if you are not ready to diet and you don't want to make any big changes, you can use your journal to add a small lifestyle goal—like reducing sodas or adding 10 minutes of exercise every day. Remember the important thing is, "Progress not Perfection"—a saying that is especially true when dieting. You don't want to wait to begin DASH and then find, when you're finally ready to diet, that you've gained five more pounds without even realizing it. Keeping a journal even if you're not yet following DASH, can help you avoid those kinds of unwanted surprises.

If you aren't ready to begin a diet now, you can use your journal to prevent further weight gain.

A Practical and Interactive Guide to DASH

The DASH Diet Solution and 60 Day Weight less and Fitness Journal is a practical and interactive diet guide designed to help you understand why you gained weight in the past, how you can replace harmful habits with positive ones now, and how to motivate and reward your dieting progress.

Since all change needs a starting point, Chapter 2 begins with your personal self-assessment.

Whether you're currently on a diet or not, try to get your calories from nutrient-rich foods.

2

My Personal Profile

What You Need to Remember:

One habit I will work to change, beginning today is:

____

1. Height: ________________

2. Weight: ________________

3. BMI (p.20): ________________

4. Lifestyle (p.27): ________________

5. Calories needed (p. 28): ________________

6. Blood Pressure*: ________________

7. Exercise, My Current Habit:

__Daily, 30-60 minutes

__Daily, 20 minutes or so

__Daily, amount of time varies

__Regularly, several days every week

__Once a week, or on the weekends only

__Sometimes a lot; other times, very little

__Almost never or never

__Other ______________________

*Many local pharmacies have machines that measure blood pressure, are easily accessed by the public and are free of charge.

8. Eating habits (check any that apply)

__snacking

__skipping meals

__sugary snacks

__salty snacks

__eating while doing other things (phone, television, reading, etc.)

__ crash diets

__ yo-yo weight—lose and gain

__ other: ______________________

9. Places where it is easy for you to make poor food choices:

___ home

___ mealtime

___ at work

___ at school

___ out with family or friends

___ other: ______________________

10. Is there any time of day that you are more likely to make bad choices?

___ morning

___ lunchtime

___ late afternoon; before dinner

___ dinner

___ evenings

___ late at night

11. Based on the above, what is one habit you want to change today?

____

____

____

12. In terms of diet and/or exercise, what is one thing that you do well? (e.g. avoid sugar, no fried food, vegetarian, good choices when eating out, vegetables daily, few "empty calories", etc.)

____

____

____

13. Looking back at what you checked on the previous pages, what other advice would you give yourself about diet, health, fitness or lifestyle?

____

____

____

____

____

3

Weight Loss and BMI

What You Need to Know About BMI

Body Mass Index (BMI) shows the ratio of your lean mass (bones, muscle, tissues) to your body fat.

How can I tell if I'm at a healthy weight?

Many people have a "desirable number" in their mind for their weight, the number they think they should see on the scale. But you may weigh more than you want to and still be within a statistically healthy range. To learn how your current weight corresponds with body fat, you can find your "body mass index" (BMI) on the chart in this chapter. This number, your BMI, is calculated based on your height and weight and will help you understand if you are at a normal weight according to current government health standards. For most people, BMI will also give you a fairly reliable indicator of your percent of body fat.

What is BMI?

Body Mass Index (BMI) shows the ratio of your lean mass (bones, muscle, tissues) to your body fat. It is not as precise as more complicated methods that directly measure body fat, but BMI does have a generally good correlation to more direct ways of measuring fat, like hydrostatic weighing (weighing in water) which is generally quite accurate, but requires a tank or a swimming pool. Skin calipers that measure the width of a fold of skin is another way of measuring fat, but requires special equipment. (A similar, though very crude, way to quickly estimate if you need to lose body fat is to pinch the skin underneath your arm between your thumb and forefinger. If the distance of skin between them is an inch or more, it is a good indication that you have too much body fat.)

Interpretation of BMI for Adults

A BMI chart is easy to read and will generally give you a good estimate of your percentage of body fat, even though it is not specifically individualized for gender, age or body build (small, medium or large). It also doesn't accurately reflect the BMI of someone with an unusual level of muscle mass. Still, for most people, BMI will give you a good approximation of your amount of body fat and whether it is in the "normal" range for your height.

Once you have this number—your BMI—it is a good idea to try to picture the results. For example, if you weigh 200 lbs and have 40% body fat (BMI of 40), roughly 120 lbs of your body is muscle, tissue and bone and 80 lbs is fat. If you weigh 200 lbs, but have only 10% body fat (a BMI of 10), you would have 180 lbs. of muscle, tissue and bone and only 20 lbs of fat and would be underweight. So two people could weigh the same but, based on their height, be very different in the amount of fat their bodies contain—and therefore, also be very different in their BMI and in their levels of health and fitness.

One of the most vivid examples of how losing weight changes your BMI happened on television several years ago when Oprah Winfrey lost 67 pounds. To show her audience how much fat that was, she came into the studio wearing her new size 10 jeans and pulling a red wagon with 67 lbs of animal fat piled onto it. It was a memorable way to illustrate what those extra numbers on the scale actually mean. If you would like to see what 67 pounds of fat looks like, you can see that show at "Oprah" online: `http://www.oprah.com/oprahshow/Oprahs-Top-20-Moments` or go to `www.oprah.com`, and then go to "Oprah's Top 20 Moments"

Norms for BMI

Use the Adult Body Mass Index (BMI) chart on the next page to see if you are underweight, at a healthy weight, overweight, or obese, then look at the categories on this page.

For adults 20 years old and older, BMI uses standard categories that are the same for all ages and for both men and women. Children and teens need to use a different chart that is age- and sex-specific.

Understanding Your BMI

BMI	**Weight Category**
Below 18.5	Underweight
18.5 – 24.9	Normal
25.0 – 29.9	Overweight
30.0 and Above	Obese

- **Underweight. If your BMI is less than 18.5**, it falls within the "underweight" range.
- **Normal weight. If your BMI is 18.5 to 24.9**, it falls within the "normal" or Healthy Weight range.
- **Overweight. If your BMI is 25.0 to 29.9**, it falls within the "overweight" range.
- **Obese. If your BMI is 30.0 or higher**, it falls within the "obese" range.

Body Mass Index Chart

Body Mass Index (BMI) Find your height, then your weight, then your BMI

	Normal						Overweight					Obese										Extreme Obesity														
BMI	19	20	21	22	23	24	25	26	27	28	29	30	31	32	33	34	35	36	37	38	39	40	41	42	43	44	45	46	47	48	49	50	51	52	53	54
Height (inches)	Body Weight (pounds)																																			
58	91	96	100	105	110	115	119	124	129	134	138	143	148	153	158	162	167	172	177	181	186	191	196	201	205	210	215	220	224	229	234	239	244	248	253	258
59	94	99	104	109	114	119	124	128	133	138	143	148	153	158	163	168	173	178	183	188	193	198	203	208	212	217	222	227	232	237	242	247	252	257	262	267
60	97	102	107	112	118	123	128	133	138	143	148	153	158	163	168	174	179	184	189	194	199	204	209	215	220	225	230	235	240	245	250	255	261	266	271	276
61	100	106	111	116	122	127	132	137	143	148	153	158	164	169	174	180	185	190	195	201	206	211	217	222	227	232	238	243	248	254	259	264	269	275	280	285
62	104	109	115	120	126	131	136	142	147	153	158	164	169	175	180	186	191	196	202	207	213	218	224	229	235	240	246	251	256	262	267	273	278	284	289	295
63	107	113	118	124	130	135	141	146	152	158	163	169	175	180	186	191	197	203	208	214	220	225	231	237	242	248	254	259	265	270	278	282	287	293	299	304
64	110	116	122	128	134	140	145	151	157	163	169	174	180	186	192	197	204	209	215	221	227	232	238	244	250	256	262	267	273	279	285	291	296	302	308	314
65	114	120	126	132	138	144	150	156	162	168	174	180	186	192	198	204	210	216	222	228	234	240	246	252	258	264	270	276	282	288	294	300	306	312	318	324
66	118	124	130	136	142	148	155	161	167	173	179	186	192	198	204	210	216	223	229	235	241	247	253	260	266	272	278	284	291	297	303	309	315	322	328	334
67	121	127	134	140	146	153	159	166	172	178	185	191	198	204	211	217	223	230	236	242	249	255	261	268	274	280	287	293	299	306	312	319	325	331	338	344
68	125	131	138	144	151	158	164	171	177	184	190	197	203	210	216	223	230	236	243	249	256	262	269	276	282	289	295	302	308	315	322	328	335	341	348	354
69	128	135	142	149	155	162	169	176	182	189	196	203	209	216	223	230	236	243	250	257	263	270	277	284	291	297	304	311	318	324	331	338	345	351	358	365
70	132	139	146	153	160	167	174	181	188	195	202	209	216	222	229	236	243	250	257	264	271	278	285	292	299	306	313	320	327	334	341	348	355	362	369	376
71	136	143	150	157	165	172	179	186	193	200	208	215	222	229	236	243	250	257	265	272	279	286	293	301	308	315	322	329	338	343	351	358	365	372	379	386
72	140	147	154	162	169	177	184	191	199	206	213	221	228	235	242	250	258	265	272	279	287	294	302	309	316	324	331	338	346	353	361	368	375	383	390	397
73	144	151	159	166	174	182	189	197	204	212	219	227	235	242	250	257	265	272	280	288	295	302	310	318	325	333	340	348	355	363	371	378	386	393	401	408
74	148	155	163	171	179	186	194	202	210	218	225	233	241	249	256	264	272	280	287	295	303	311	319	326	334	342	350	358	365	373	381	389	396	404	412	420
75	152	160	168	176	184	192	200	208	216	224	232	240	248	256	264	272	279	287	295	303	311	319	327	335	343	351	359	367	375	383	391	399	407	415	423	431
76	156	164	172	180	189	197	205	213	221	230	238	246	254	263	271	279	287	295	304	312	320	328	336	344	353	361	369	377	385	394	402	410	418	426	435	443

Date: ____________________

My Weight is: ___________

My Height is: ___________

My BMI is: ___________

Knowing Your Healthy Weight

"Underweight", "normal", "overweight", and "obese" are all labels for ranges of weight. “Obese” and “overweight” describe ranges of weight that are greater than what is considered healthy for a given height, while “underweight” describes a weight that is lower than is generally healthy.

BMI is good to know, but if you feel that your “normal” weight according to the chart is still heavier than you feel is right for your body, you can look at the range of healthy weights for your height. You may be at the upper range now and be glad to know that you are statistically within a healthy range. But, knowing your own body—and in consultation with your doctor—you may feel that you are more fit at the lower part of healthy BMI weight range and can choose that target weight instead.

For example, a woman who is 5’8” tall and 155 pounds is within the healthy range on the BMI chart. But she may feel that she looks and feels better at 140 lbs, which is also a healthy weight for that height, according to BMI. So BMI is a range within which you should aim for good health, and then make a judgment related to your own fitness and appearance.

BMI if You are Athletic

According to the American Council on Exercise, an athletic woman typically has 14 to 20 percent body fat, and athletic men have 6 to 13 percent. For a “fit” woman, the range is 21 to 24 percent while fit men are 14 to 17 percent.

BMI is used as a screening method, but a health care professional is the best person to evaluate your overall health and fitness.

Overweight and Obesity

BMI defines "overweight" as a body mass index of 25 or higher, and "obesity" is categorized as a BMI of 30 or higher. Overweight and obesity can both contribute to serious health problems, including heart disease, diabetes, stroke and cancer. Conversely, good nutrition and exercise—combined with maintaining a healthy weight—may delay or prevent the onset of disease, slow the affects of aging, and reduce your risk factors for numerous illnesses. Studies of healthy diets from Greece to Okinawa have supported the idea that regularly eating nutrient-rich fruits and vegetables and generally avoiding animal fats can help your immune system, reduce the effects of aging and increase life expectancy.

The key to achieving and maintaining a healthy weight isn't about quick fixes and short-term dietary changes. It's about building a lifestyle that includes healthy eating, regular physical activity, and balancing the number of calories you consume with the number of calories that your body uses.

For overweight or obese adults, it is beneficial to lose even a small amount of weight.

If you are overweight and are not dieting, it is particularly important to be sure you are not gaining more weight.

4

The Calorie Balance

What You Need to Remember About Calories
3500 calories = 1 pound of body weight

What is a Calorie?

Nearly every diet mentions calories. But what is a calorie? Scientifically speaking, a calorie is defined as the amount of heat that is needed to raise 1 gram of water by 1° Celsius (the equivalent of 4.1840 joules.)

Nutritionally speaking, a calorie is a unit of energy that is produced by food.

When it comes to maintaining a healthy weight for a lifetime, the bottom line is – **calories count!** Weight management is all about balance—balancing the number of calories you consume with the number of calories your body uses or "burns off."

- **A *calorie* is defined as a unit of energy supplied by food.** A calorie is a calorie regardless of its source. Whether you're eating carbohydrates, fats, sugars, or proteins, all of them contain calories.
- ***Caloric balance* is like a scale.** To remain in balance and maintain your body weight, the calories consumed (from foods) must be balanced by the calories used (in normal body functions, daily activities, and exercise).

> **"How many calories are there per gram?"**
>
> **protein = 4 calories per gram**
> **carbohydrate = 4 calories per gram**
> **fat = 9 calories per gram**

Protein, fats, and carbohydrates all contain calories. Interestingly, your metabolism of a protein or carbohydrate produces approximately 4 calories for each gram, but metabolizing a gram of fat is more than double that—nearly 9 calories for each gram of fat your body consumes. This helps explain the continuing popularity of high protein, low fat diets.

In 1990, the U.S. Food and Drug Administration began requiring calories to be listed on all food labels. By understanding your own caloric needs and remaining aware of the calories in the food you eat, you can get into what's known as caloric balance and help yourself achieve and maintain a healthy weight.

Am I in Caloric Balance?

If you are maintaining your current body weight, you are in caloric balance. If you need to gain weight or to lose weight, you'll need to tip the balance scale in one direction or another to reach your goal.

Remember, each pound represents 3,500 calories. If you reduce your calories 500-1000 a day, you can lose 1 or 2 pounds a week.

My Weight Loss Timetable

1. I want to lose ________________ pounds.
2. If I lose 2 lbs a week, it will take me ____ weeks. (pounds ÷ 2/week)
3. This means reducing my calories by ______ a week or _____ a day.

For example: 1. You want to lose 20 lbs 2. It will take 10 weeks 3. You need to take in 7000 calories less a week, or 1000 fewer calories a day. You can see from this example, how difficult it is to lose weight by diet alone, and how important exercise is in helping acheive weight loss.

What are my Calorie Needs?

The number of calories you need depends on how much energy your body uses. This is based on many things including your gender, age, weight, and activity level. You may suffer negative physical consequences, like rapid hair loss, from consuming too few calories or become obese from consuming too many. In dieting, as in so many things, balance is the key. When your body takes in the number of calories it uses, you will be maintaining your optimum weight. Calorie balance, combined with good nutrition, will mean that you have achieved an optimum weight that is also your healthy weight. To lose weight, you need a sustained calorie deficit over time, but in a way that maintains your health. DASH can do this. That's why, in addition to "#1 Diabetes Diet" and "#1 Best Overall Die"t, *U.S. News and World Report* also named DASH as the "#1 Diet for Healthy Eating".

"Low-fat" doesn't mean "low calorie"

Now that you know that every gram of fat has nearly twice as many calories as a gram of carbohydrate or protein, you can understand the appeal of low-fat diets. Many people think that by eliminating the high calorie count of a gram of fat, they will easily lose weight with a low-fat diet. However, it is important to remember that just because a food is low-fat does not mean it is necessarily also low in calories. For example, that large bran muffin at the local coffee shop may say "low-fat" on the label, but still contain over 400 calories of eggs, flour, fat, sugar and other calorie-producing ingredients. "Low fat" foods can still be high in calories and you can still find yourself gaining weight from eating them. This is one reason why it is important to read the nutrition information.

For many years, the U.S. government has required nutrition information, including calories, on the packaged food that's sold in supermarkets. But it is only since 2011 that fast food chains and restaurants have also been required to display their menu's nutrition content. The legislated regulations vary from state to state, with California having the strictest standards. But all states are now required to have some way of showing customers the calorie count of the food they eat. Studies have shown that when people can see the nutrition content—especially calories, fat, sugar and salt—they will make healthier food choices.

3500 calories = 1 pound of body weight

If you want to lose weight, you need to consume fewer calories than your body needs. To lose 1 pound of body weight, you need to reduce your calories to 3,500 calories less than your body uses. The best way to do this, of course, is to burn more calories than you need by increasing your activity level and decreasing your calories. You can do this easily with DASH, creating a calorie deficit and losing weight without compromising your health and energy.

Are Your Calories in Balance?

If you are...	Your caloric balance status is...
Maintaining your weight	"**in balance**." You are eating the same number of calories that your body is using. Your weight will remain **stable**.
Gaining weight	"**in caloric excess**." You are eating more calories than your body uses. You store these extra calories as fat and gain weight.
Losing weight	"**in caloric deficit**." You are eating fewer calories than you are using. Your body is pulling from fat storage cells.

The number of servings you'll need for each food group in the DASH Diet depends, of course, on the number of calories you're allowed each day. Your calorie level depends most of all on how active you are. Think of this as an energy balance system—if you want to maintain your current weight, you should take in only as many calories as you use. If you need to lose weight, eat fewer calories than you burn and/or increase your activity level to burn more calories than you consume.

Eat fewer calories than you burn or increase your activity level so that you burn more calories than you consume.

Remember, it is always important to eat foods that are high in nutrients for the amount of calories they contain, such as vegetables, fruits, whole grains, and low-fat or fat free dairy products.. And don't forget to watch your portion size. Controlling portion size helps limit calorie intake, especially when eating foods that are high in calories.

To lose weight, you need to understand the relationship between your calorie intake and your activity level. Read the descriptions below and check the category that best describes your typical daily activity level.

What's Your Lifestyle?: Activity Level Chart (check one)

__**Sedentary** – a lifestyle that includes only the light physical activity associated with typical day-to-day life.

__**Moderately active** – a lifestyle that includes physical activity equivalent to walking about 1.5 to 3 miles per day at 3 to 4 miles per hour, in addition to the light physical activity associated with typical day-to-day life.

__**Active** – a lifestyle that includes physical activity equivalent to walking more than 3 miles per day at 3 to4 miles per hour, in addition to the light physical activity associated with typical day-to-day life.

My usual activity level is

__**Sedentary** __**Moderately active** __**Active**

My daily calories should be: ____________________

(See calorie chart on page 28.)

How Many Calories Do You Need?
Based on Gender, Age, and Activity Level

Gender	Age/Yrs.	Calories		
		Sedentary	**Moderately Active**	**Active**
Child	2 – 3	1,000	1,000 - 1,400	1,000 - 1,400
Female	4 – 8	1,200	1,400 - 1,600	1,400 - 1,800
	9 – 13	1,600	1,600 - 2,000	1,800 - 2,200
	14 – 18	1,800	2,000	2,400
	19 – 30	2,000	2,000 - 2,200	2,400
	31 – 50	1,800	2,000	2,400
	51+	1,600	1,800	2,000 - 2,200
Male	4 – 8	1,400	1,400 - 1,600	1,600 - 2,000
	9 – 13	1,800	1,800 - 2,200	2,000 - 2,600
	14 – 18	2,200	2,400 - 2,800	2,800 - 3,200
	19 – 30	2,400	2,600 - 2,800	3,000
	31 – 50	2,200	2,400 - 2,600	2,800 - 3,000
	51+	2,000	2,200 - 2,400	2,400 - 2,800

Calorie Ranges. The calorie ranges shown are to accommodate needs of different ages within the group. For adults, fewer calories are needed at older ages. For more information on the *Dietary Guidelines for Americans*, go online to:

www.healthierus.gov/dietaryguidelines.

These levels are based on Estimated Energy Requirements (EER) from the Institute of Medicine (IOM) Dietary Reference Intakes macro-nutrients report,2002, calculated by gender, age, and activity level for reference-sized individuals. "Reference size," as determined by IOM, is based on median height and weightfor ages up to age 18 years of age and median height and weight for that height to give a Body Mass Index(BMI) of 21.5 for adult females and 22.5 for adult males.

How to Replace High Calorie Food with Lower Calorie Food

The DASH Diet promotes weight loss. It is rich in lower-calorie foods, such as fruits and vegetables. You can make it even lower in calories by replacing higher calorie foods, such as sweets, with more fruits and vegetables, and that also will make it easier for you to reach your DASH goals. Here are some examples of how a few easy changes can add up to calorie savings.

Fruit. To increase fruits, have...

- **a medium apple** instead of four shortbread cookies.

  You'll save 80 calories.

- **dried apricots** (1/4 cup) instead of a 2-ounce bag of pork rinds.

  You'll save 230 calories.

Vegetables and Protein. To increase vegetables, have...

- **a hamburger** that's 3 ounces of meat instead of 6 ounces. Add a serving of carrots (1/2 cup) and a serving of spinach (1/2 cup).

  You'll save more than 200 calories.

- **Stir fry.** Instead of 5 ounces of chicken, have a stir fry with 2 ounces of chicken and 1½ cups of raw vegetables. Use a small amount of vegetable oil.

  You'll save 50 calories

Dairy. To increase low-fat milk products, have...

- **low-fat frozen yogurt** (1/2 cup) instead of a 1/2-cup serving of full-fat ice cream.

  You'll save about 70 calories.

Remember these calorie-saving tips:

- Choose fat-free or low-fat condiments.
- Use half as much vegetable oil, soft or liquid margarine, mayonnaise, or salad dressing, or choose available low-fat or fat-free versions.
- Eat smaller portions—cut back gradually.
- Choose fat-free or low-fat milk and milk products.
- Limit foods with lots of added sugar, such as pies, flavored yogurts, candy bars, ice cream, sherbet, regular soft drinks, and fruit drinks.
- Eat fruits canned in their own juice or in water.
- Add fruit to plain fat-free or low-fat yogurt.
- Snack on fruit, vegetable sticks, unbuttered and unsalted popcorn, or rice cakes.
- Drink water or club soda—zest it up with a wedge of lemon or lime.

Now choose one of the tips on the list above to add to your own lifestyle. I will

____

____

Remember, for a Healthy Diet:

- Make smart choices from every food group.
- Find balance between food and physical activity.
- Get the most nutrition out of calories.
- Stay within your daily calorie needs

Staying in control of your weight contributes to good health now and as you age.

5

Salt: Is it Hazardous to Your Health?

What You Need to Remember About Sodium

1500 mg of sodium is roughly ¾ tsp. of salt.
2300 mg of sodium is roughly 1 tsp. of salt.

As you read in Chapter 1, the DASH Diet began as the National Health Institute's research to fight high blood pressure, but the results of the studies exceeded the researchers' expectations. Not only did participants who followed DASH succeed in lowering their blood pressure, they also lost a significant amount of weight and improved their health.

What is High Blood Pressure?

When blood circulates through your body, it presses against the artery walls. The amount of force it exerts is measured as blood pressure.

Blood pressure is measured in millimeters of mercury (mm/Hg) and is recorded as two numbers. For example, a blood pressure measurement of 120/80 mmHg (millimeters of mercury) is expressed verbally as "120 over 80." The systolic pressure, the top number, is the blood pressure as the heart beats. The bottom number is called the diastolic pressure and measures the pressure as the heart relaxes between beats. Normal blood pressure is less than 120 mmHg for the systolic measurement, and less than 80 mmHg for the diastolic.

Blood pressure can be influenced by many factors, and it typically rises and falls throughout the day. If it stays high over time, it can cause serious health problems, including an increased risk for heart disease, the leading cause of death in the United States.

When blood pressure is consistently high, the heart has to work harder. The pressure of the circulating blood can also harm arteries and vital organs. High blood pressure can lead to kidney and heart disease, stroke and blindness.

High blood pressure is often called the "silent killer" because it has no warning signs and many people, including young adults, don't realize they have it. It affects 1 in 3 Americans--more than 65 million people in the U.S. and over 1 billion people globally. An additional 28 percent of adult Americans have prehypertension.

High blood pressure is even more common among African Americans, and it tends to develop earlier for them than for other groups. Hypertension is also common for older Americans. Even if you have normal blood pressure when you're 55, you have a 90 percent chance of developing high blood pressure in your lifetime.

There is a clear relationship between your salt intake and your blood pressure. When you significantly decrease your salt consumption, you will see the resulting lower blood pressure, often within only two weeks. People with high blood pressure and prehypertension may especially benefit from following the DASH eating plan and reducing their sodium intake. If your blood pressure is currently normal, the DASH diet can help you keep it that way.

If you already have hypertension, you should be able to see benefits quite quickly when you follow DASH and reduce your sodium. According to the Center for Disease Control (CDC), even a small change in salt consumption—like reducing daily sodium by 400 mg (less than ¼ of a teaspoon)—could save 28,000 lives a year.

90% of adult Americans eat too much salt.

What is Your Blood Pressure?

Blood Pressure Chart

Normal

Less than 120 diastolic *and*
Less than 80 systolic < 120/80

Prehypertension

120–139 diastolic *or*
80–89 systolic

Hypertension

140 or higher diastolic *or*
90 or higher

Date: ____________

My blood pressure is: ___________

This number means that my blood pressure is:

__ Normal __Prehypertension __ Hypertension

The Typical American Diet is High in Sodium

The DASH menus in this book have 2,300 milligrams of sodium—much lower than the typical American diet—and each one shows how easily you can modify them to have only 1,500 milligrams of sodium. This is much lower than the typical American diet, since some reports estimate that the average American women consumes about 3,300 milligrams of sodium per day, while men get about 4,200 milligrams daily.

44% of the Sodium in the typical American diet comes from only 10 foods

Nearly 90% of American adults eat too much salt. According to the CDC, most of this unneeded sodium comes from the food we buy in restaurants and supermarkets.

A surprising 2012 study from the Center for Disease Control revealed that bread and rolls, not salty snacks, are the main source of sodium in the typical American's diet. This is not because bread is especially high in salt, but because bread is such a dietary staple in the United States.

How Many of These Foods Do You Routinely Have?

Here is the list of the ten foods that account for nearly half of the salt that Americans typically eat every day. To get an idea of your own consumption of these foods, put a (D) next to items you eat Daily, a (W) for those you have Weekly, and an (M) for any that you have monthly. Mark food that you rarely eat with (R) or an (N) for Never. See if these foods are as common for you as they are for most Americans.

___ 1. breads and rolls

___ 2. meat dishes (meatloaf, meatballs, etc.)

___ 3. poultry dishes or as processed food

___ 4. pizza

___ 5. cheeseburgers and other sandwiches

___ 6. cheese

___ 7. pasta dishes

___ 8. soup

___ 9. cold cuts like ham and turkey

___10, snack foods including chips, pretzels, and popcorn

Based on the high-sodium foods I checked above, I will begin to eat less of this:

____

____

Sodium and Processed Foods

Most of the sodium we eat comes from packaged, processed, store-bought, and restaurants foods. Only a small amount comes from salt added during cooking or at the dining table. Over-salted processed foods are so commonplace for people in the United States that most Americans have already exceeded their daily limit of sodium before they evem sit down for dinner—sometimes, even before lunch.

If you want to reduce sodium, it is best to buy fresh and fresh-frozen produce. One caution about buying packaged (canned, dried, or frozen) fruits and vegetables is that, in addition to high quantities of sodium, they may contain added sugars or saturated fats. These are also ingredients that you will want to look for and to limit.

For these reasons, it is important to read the labels of the packaged food you buy in markets. There is a lot of good information there and some of it can be very unexpected. For example, many people are surprised to learn that a common diet food like cottage cheese is quite high in sodium.

Where to Find Ingredients on a Package

There are three places to look for ingredients on a package and they each give important information about the product:

- the ingredient list
- the Nutrition Facts label, and
- the front label of the package.

Read the Nutrition Label

By law, products are required to have nutrition labels and they are filled with useful information. Read the Nutrition Facts labels on different brands of food to compare the amount of sodium, potassium and other nutrients in packaged products. The sodium content is listed in milligrams and the label will list it as the percent of Daily Value (%DV) that is considered safe to consume.

Nutrition Facts Label: an Example

Nutrition Facts		
Serving Size	1/2 cup (4 oz.)	
Servings Per Container 2		
Amount Per Serving		
Calories 250	Calories from Fat 110	
% Daily Value*		
Total Fat	12g	18%
Saturated Fat	3g	15%
Trans Fat	3g	
Cholesterol	30mg	10%
Sodium	470mg	20%
Potassium	7 00mg	20%
Total Carbohydrate	31g	10%
Dietary Fiber	5g	20%
Sugars	5g	
Protein	5g	

Reading a label. Above is an example of a Nutrition Facts label for a carton of yogurt.

How many calories are there in the carton? ________

What is the serving size? ________

How many calories are there per serving? ________

Answers: 1. 500 calories. 2. ½ cup 3. 250 calories. When you see the serving size is ½ cup and the calories are 250 per serving, you know that the entire carton of yogurt is 2 servings, or 500 calories for 8 ounces. This kind of information is especially important to look for on desserts and other fat- and sugar-laden foods. The calorie count on a package of cookies, for example, may seem low—until you read that it is 100 calories for a serving of only two cookies.

Look at the chart below to see if there are foods you need to limit in your current diet.

Sodium Content (mg)
% Daily Value (DV)

	Sodium Content (mg)	(% DV)*
Breads, all types 1 oz	95 - 210	4%
Frozen pizza, plain cheese 4 oz	450 - 1,200	19% - 50%
Frozen vegetables, all types 1/2 c	2 - 160	0% - 7%
Salad dressing, 2 Tbsp (reg.fat)	110 - 505	5% - 21%
Salsa 2 Tbsp	150 - 240	6% - 10%
Soup (tomato), reconstituted 8 oz	700 - 1,260	29% - 53%
Tomato juice 8 oz (~1 c)	340 - 1,040	14% - 43%
Potato chips 1 oz (28.4 g)	120 - 180	5% - 8%
Tortilla chips 1 oz (28.4 g)	105 - 160	4% - 7%
Pretzels[a] 1 oz (28.4 g)	290 - 560	12% - 23%

Source for Sodium Chart: *Serving sizes were standardized to be comparable among brands within a food. Pizza and bread slices vary in size and weight across brands.Note: None of the examples provided were labeled low-sodium products.* % Daily Values (DV) listed in this column are based on the food amounts listed in the table. The DV for sodium is 2,400 mg.*

[a] *All snack foods are regular flavor, salted. Source: Agriculture Research Service (ARS) Nutrient Database for Standard Reference, Release 17 and recent manufacturers' label data from retail market surveys.*

High sodium foods I want to cut back on or avoid

Using the list on the previous page or other lists of salty foods in this chapter, are there any high-sodium foods that you need to reduce or eliminate completely from your current diet? Write any of them down in the space below. Also remember to look for flavorful low salt (or better yet, no salt) alternatives for your favorite snack foods.

Not All Canned Products are the Same

Compare the food labels of two kinds of canned tomatoes below and on the next page. Is the difference in sodium content significant?

Nutrition Facts

Low Sodium Canned Diced Tomatoes

Serving Size 1/2 cup (130g)
Servings Per Container 31/2

Amount Per Serving	
Calories 25	Calories from Fat 0
	% Daily Value*
Total Fat	0g **0%**
Saturated Fat	0g **0%**
***Trans* Fat**	0g **0%**
Cholesterol	0mg **0%**
Sodium	10mg **1%**
Potassium	270mg **8%**
Total Carbohydrate	5g **2%**
Dietary Fiber	1g **4%**
Sugar 3g	
Protein 1g	
Vitamin A 5%	**Vitamin C** 30%
Calcium 4%	**Iron** 4%

**Percent Daily Values are based on a 2,000 calorie diet.*

In the example below, you can see how useful a nutrition label is. It is easy to use the Daily Value listing (% DV) on it to look for foods that are low in sodium. You can also look for potassium on nutrition labels. Although not all labels list it, many do. When possible, it is a good idea to choose products that are high in potassium since it counteracts some of sodium's negative effects on blood pressure. (You can read more about potassium in Ch 6.)

Aim for foods that contain 5 percent or less of the Daily Value of sodium. Foods with 20 percent or more Daily Value (DV) of sodium are considered high. These include baked goods, certain cereals, soy sauce, and some antacids.

Nutrition Facts

Canned Diced Tomatoes

Serving Size 1/2 cup (130g)
Servings Per Container 3 ½

Amount Per Serving	
Calories 25	Calories from Fat 0
	% Daily Value*
Total Fat	0g **0%**
Saturated Fat	0g **0%**
***Trans* Fat**	0g **0%**
Cholesterol	0mg **0%**
Sodium	150mg **6%**
Potassium	270mg **8%**
Total Carbohydrate	5g **2%**
Dietary Fiber	1g **4%**
Sugar 3g	
Protein 1g	
Vitamin A 5%	**Vitamin C** 30%
Calcium 4%	**Iron** 4%

**Percent Daily Values are based on a 2,000 calorie diet.*

Understanding Nutrition Facts Label and Daily Value (% DV)

The nutrition labels on the previous pages show that a half a cup of the regular canned tomatoes has 15 times as much sodium as the low-sodium canned tomatoes. If you had to choose between the two, one cup of regular canned tomatoes has 300 mg of sodium, while a cup of low-sodium tomatoes has 20 mg. From this comparison, you can see how easy it is to make food choices throughout the day that add large amounts of sodium to your diet without even realizing it.

Alternatives to salt. Instead of adding salt to food, be creative. Experiment with:

herbs	spices
lemon	lime
vinegar	wine
salt-free seasoning blends	

Since most sodium is found in processed food, it is good to know the different ways it can be listed on the label and what each listing means.

Terms for Low Sodium

Sodium free or salt free

Very low sodium

Low sodium

Reduced or less sodium

Light in sodium

Unsalted or no salt added

Understanding Label Language: Sodium

Sodium	What it Means*
Sodium free or salt free	Less than 5 mg per serving
Very low sodium	35 mg or less of sodium per serving
Low sodium	140 mg or less of sodium per serving
Low-sodium meal	140 mg or less of sodium per 31/2 oz (100 g)
Reduced or less sodium	At least 25 percent less sodium than the regular version
Light in sodium	50 percent less sodium than the regular version
Unsalted or no salt added	No salt added to the product during processing (this is not a sodium-free food)

Only a small amount of sodium occurs naturally in food. Most sodium is added during processing.

4 Ways to Reduce Sodium When Eating Out

- Ask how foods are prepared. Ask that they be prepared without added salt, MSG, or salt-containing ingredients. Most restaurants are willing to accommodate requests.
- Know the terms that indicate high sodium content: pickled, cured, smoked, soy sauce, broth.
- Move the salt shaker away.
- Limit condiments, such as mustard, ketchup, pickles, and sauces with salt-containing ingredients. Start by cutting salt in half.

Public Disclosure in Restaurants. Also remember that restaurants and fast food chains must now post nutrition information, including the sodium content of their food. Check this information before ordering; you may be surprised at the high-sodium entrees and what is low in salt.

Ways to Eat Less Salt

Check anything on this list that you will begin doing

___ 1. **Nutrition Facts label.** Check the sodium content on it.

___ 2. **Daily Value (% DV).** Use the percent Daily Value (% DV) to judge my sodium intake for the day.

___ 3. **Compare sodium content** for similar foods.

___ 4. **Use herbs and spices** at home to add flavor instead of salt.

___ 5. **Don't salt foods** before or during cooking.

___ 6. **Ask restaurants** to not salt my food.

___ 7. **Choose condiments** that are low-sodium or no-salt added when available. Limit low sodium soy sauce and teriyaki

___ 8. **Use fresh meats**—poultry, fish, beef and pork, rather than canned, smoked, or processed types.

___ 9 **Choose cereal** that is lower in salt.

___ 10. **Avoid cured foods** (bacon, hot dogs), brine-packed foods (olives,sauerkraut, pickles), condiments (mustard, horseradish,ketchup).

___ 11. **Cook without salt** when I make rice, pasta or cereal.

___ 12. **Cut back on processed foods**—like canned foods and frozen dinners high in sodium (that is most of them).

___ 13. **Rinse canned food** like tuna and beans to reduce the salt.

Recommended Sodium %DV on Processed Food Labels

Look for 5% DV for Sodium
Avoid 20% Daily Value (DV) of Sodium.

If you follow the tips in this chapter, in a short time, your taste for salt will decrease, and you won't miss it.

6

"Am I Getting Enough Potassium?"

What You Need to Remember
For most people, the daily Potassium Goal should be 4700 mg

Why Potassium?

A potassium-rich diet can help to reduce elevated or high blood pressure. Most people should aim for 4700 mg per day; be sure to get your potassium from food sources, not from supplements, if possible.

Many fruits and vegetables, some milk products, and fish are all rich sources of potassium. However, fruits and vegetables are rich in the form of potassium (potassium with bicarbonate precursors) that favorably affects acid-base metabolism.

The DASH Diet plan emphasizes potassium from food, especially fruits and vegetables, to help keep blood pressure levels healthy.

In the last chapter, you read about some of the health problems that sodium creates. You also saw some of the common foods it is found in (mostly, it is in processed foods). If you used the spaces provided to write reminder notes about salty foods you want to avoid or at least cut back on, you already have the beginnings of a DASH dietary action plan.

In this chapter, you will look at potassium, but with the opposite goal from Chapter 4. Unlike sodium, potassium is good for you. The challenge with potassium is to get enough of it—and, preferably, to get it from natural foods rather than from supplements.

Your goal is to get about 4700 mg. of potassium every day. As you can see from the chart on the next page, this can take a bit of planning.

Potassium-rich Foods

Ways to Include Potassium in Your Diet

	Potassium (mg)	% Daily Value*	Calories
Sweet potato, baked 1 (146 g)	694	20%	131
Beet greens, cooked, 1/2 c	655	19%	19
Potato, baked, flesh, 1 potato	610	17%	145
White beans, canned, 1/2 c	595	17%	153
Yogurt, plain, non-fat, 8-oz	579	17%	127
Clams, canned, 3 oz	534	15%	126
Yogurt, plain, low-fat, 8-oz	531	15%	143
Prune juice, 3/4 c	530	15%	136
Carrot juice, 3/4 c	517	14%	71
Halibut, cooked, 3 oz	490	14%	119
Soybeans, green, cooked, 1/2 c	485	14%	127
Tuna, yellowfin, cooked, 3 oz	484	14%	118
Lima beans, cooked, 1/2 c	484	14%	104
Winter squash, cooked, 1/2 c	448	13%	40
Soybeans, mature, cooked, 1/2 c	443	13%	149
Rockfish, Pacific, cooked, 3 oz	442	13%	103
Cod, Pacific, cooked, 3 oz	439	13%	89
Banana, 1 medium	422	12%	105
Spinach, cooked, 1/2 c	419	12%	21
Tomato juice, 3/4 c	417	12%	31
Tomato sauce, 1/2 c	405	12%	39

Source: Nutrient values from Agricultural Research Service (ARS) Nutrient Database for Standard Reference, Release 17.Foods are from ARS single nutrient reports, sorted in descending order by nutrient content in terms of common householdmeasures. Food items and weights in the single nutrient reports are adapted from those in 2002 revision of USDA Home and Garden Bulletin No. 72, Nutritive Value of Foods. Mixed dishes and multiple preparations of the same food item have been omitted from this table. For more information on the *Dietary Guidelines for Americans*, please visit www.healthierus.gov/dietaryguidelines.

Other good sources of Potassium are:

- **Dried fruits** (various) – ½ of raisins has 540 mg. (Get pesticide-free ones though.)
- **Oranges** – an 8 oz. glass of orange juice has 480 mg.
- **Cantaloupe**, and honeydew melons – ½ cup has 490 mg.
- **Tomato products** – 6 oz. of tomato juice has 650 mg.
- **Dates** – a ¼ cup has 584 mg
- **Avocado** – ½ avocado has 490 mg
- **Milk** – 1 cup has 380 mg. Aim for low- or non-fat.

As you can see, you could meet your goal with 1 baked sweet potato (700 mg), 1/2 cup of canned white beans (600 mg), 1 cup of plain yogurt (580 mg), 3/4 cup of prune juice (530 mg), 3/4 cup of carrot juice (520 mg), 6 oz of cooked halibut (900 mg) and 1 banana (420 mg), but as you can see, it takes some planning. The typical idea of "I'll just have a banana" meets less than a tenth of your daily potassium need.

Luckily, many common foods also have potassium, just at lower levels (3 oz. of ground beef has 220 mg) so most people will get some potassium daily easily and not have to plan carefully for all of it. But, as you can see, for most people it will be necessary to make a conscious effort to boost your potassium consumption—whether by increasing servings of non-fat yogurt and milk, adding a sweet potato, routinely adding avocado to your salads, making a potassium-rich smoothie with fruit, or having a glass of orange juice or tomato juice every day. Also remember that three cups of non-fat milk or yogurt easily adds 1000 mg of potassium a day.

Potassium-rich foods I will eat more often:

____

____

____

____

____

____

My Lifestyle Changes So Far

This is the end of the sixth chapter. By now, you have read about many ways to improve your diet or lifestyle—from small things like eating more potassium-rich foods to more difficult goals like limiting your sodium intake to 1500 mg. a day, or cutting calories by 500-1000 calories a day. But have you really made any changes yet?

Yes, I have already made a change. Now I ____________________

____

If you haven 't made a change yet, look back over the past chapters and choose a goal. There have been many suggestions. Choose something new to do daily to improve your lifestyle.

Beginning today, I will choose to ____________________________

____

____

____

____

____

____

____

____

____

For example: *"Beginning today, I will choose to have a non-fat latte with no sweetner and a banana instead of a regular latte with a low-fat muffin. This will help me by reducing my calories and improving my daily potassium intake."*

Or, *"Beginning today, I will exercise for at least 20 minutes and eat the number of servings of fruits and vegetables required on DASH."*

7
Good or Bad Fat?

What You Need to Know
Eat less saturated fat, trans fat, and cholesterol.
It is important to eat less than 10%
of your calories from saturated fat.

Know Your Fats

The good news is that there *is* such a thing as "good fat". Fats and oils are part of a healthy diet and play many important roles in the body. Fat provides energy and is a carrier of essential nutrients such as vitamins A, D, E, K, and carotenoids. But, fat can impact the health of your heart and arteries in a positive or negative way, depending on the types of fat you eat. DASH limits your daily fats, so choose wisely.

Foods can contain a mixture of different fats. Unsaturated fats are considered "good" fats. They're sometimes listed as "monounsaturated" and "polyunsaturated" fat on Nutrition Facts labels. These can promote health if eaten in the right amounts. They are generally liquid at room temperature. You'll find healthful unsaturated fats in fish, nuts and most vegetable oils, including canola, corn, olive and safflower oils.

The so-called "bad" fats are saturated fats and trans fats. They tend to be solid at room temperature. Solid fats include butter, meat fats, stick margarine, shortening, and coconut and palm oils. They're often found in chocolates, baked goods, and deep-fried and processed foods. They can add to blood cholesterol and cause plaque to form in artery walls. This can lead to heart disease, the number one cause of death in the U.S.

The following information from NIH (National Institute of Health) will give you a good idea of what cholesterol is, why it is important and how to control it.

Why Is Cholesterol Important?

Your blood cholesterol level has a lot to do with your chances of getting heart disease. A risk factor is a condition that increases your chance of getting a disease, and high blood cholesterol is one of the major risk factors for heart disease. In fact, the higher your blood cholesterol level, the greater your risk for developing heart disease or having a heart attack. Heart disease is the number one killer of men and women in the United States. Each year, more than a million Americans have heart attacks, and about half a million people die from heart disease.

How Does Cholesterol Cause Heart Disease?

When there is too much cholesterol (a fat-like substance) in your blood, it builds up in the walls of your arteries. Over time, this buildup causes "hardening of the arteries" so that arteries become narrowed and blood flow to the heart is slowed down or blocked. The blood carries oxygen to the heart, and if enough blood and oxygen cannot reach your heart, you may suffer chest pain. If the blood supply to a portion of the heart is completely cut off by a blockage, the result is a heart attack.

High blood cholesterol itself does not cause symptoms, so many people are unaware that their cholesterol level is dangerously high. It is important to find out what your cholesterol numbers are because lowering cholesterol levels that are too high lessens the risk for developing heart disease—or of dying from it—and it reduces your chance of having a heart attack. Keeping a healthy cholesterol is important for everyone—whether you are a young, middle aged, or an older adult; male or female; with or without heart disease.

Everyone age 20 and older should have their cholesterol measured at least once every five years. You can find out your cholesterol numbers with a blood test called a "lipoprotein profile". This blood test is done after a 9- to 12-hour fast.

What Do Your Cholesterol Numbers Mean?

LDL (bad) cholesterol—This is the main source of cholesterol buildup and blockage in the arteries.

HDL (good) cholesterol—This helps keep cholesterol from building up in the arteries.

Triglycerides—This is another form of fat in your blood.

If it is not possible to get a lipoprotein profile done, knowing your total cholesterol and HDL cholesterol can give you a general idea about your cholesterol levels. If your total cholesterol is 200 mg/dL* or more or if your HDL is less than 40 mg/dL, you will need to have a lipoprotein profile done. See how your cholesterol numbers compare to the tables below.

Total Cholesterol Level	Category
Less than 200 mg/dL	Desirable
200-239 mg/dL	Borderline High
240 mg/dL and above	High

* Cholesterol levels are measured in milligrams (mg) of cholesterol per deciliter (dL) of blood.

Your Cholesterol

Date: ____________________

My Cholesterol Level: ____________________

It is (circle one): Desirable Borderline High High

LDL __________ HDL __________ Triglycerides __________

Understanding Cholesterol Levels

LDL Cholesterol Level	LDL-Cholesterol Category
Less than 100 mg/dL	Optimal
100-129 mg/dL	Near optimal/above optimal
130-159 mg/dL	Borderline high
160-189 mg/dL	High
190 mg/dL and above	Very high

HDL (good) cholesterol protects against heart disease, so for HDL, higher numbers are better. A level less than 40 mg/dL is low and is considered a major risk factor because it increases your risk for developing heart disease. HDL levels of 60 mg/dL or more help to lower your risk for heart disease.

Triglycerides can also raise heart disease risk. Levels that are borderline high (150-199 mg/dL) or high (200 mg/dL or more) may need treatment in some people.

What Affects Cholesterol Levels?

Diet. Saturated fat and cholesterol in the food you eat make your blood cholesterol level go up. Saturated fat is the main culprit, but cholesterol in foods also matters. Reducing the amount of saturated fat and cholesterol in your diet helps lower your blood cholesterol level.

Weight. Being overweight is a risk factor for heart disease. It also tends to increase your cholesterol. Losing weight can help lower your LDL and total cholesterol levels, as well as raise your HDL and lower your triglyceride levels.

Physical Activity. Not being physically active is a risk factor for heart disease. Regular physical activity can help lower LDL (bad) cholesterol and raise HDL (good) cholesterol levels. It also helps you lose weight. You should try to be physically active for 30 minutes on most days.

Things you cannot do anything about also can affect cholesterol levels. These include:

Age and Gender. As women and men get older, their cholesterol levels rise. Before the age of menopause, women have lower total cholesterol levels than men of the same age. After the age of menopause, women's LDL levels tend to rise.

Heredity. Your genes partly determine how much cholesterol your body makes. High blood cholesterol can run in families.

What Is Your Risk of Developing Heart Disease or Having a Heart Attack?

In general, the higher your LDL level and the more risk factors you have (other than LDL), the greater your chances of developing heart disease or having a heart attack. Some people are at high risk for a heart attack because they already have heart disease. Other people are at high risk for developing heart disease because they have diabetes (which is a strong risk factor) or a combination of risk factors for heart disease. Follow the steps below to find out your risk for developing heart disease.

Major Risk Factors That Affect Your LDL Goal

Step 1: Check the list below to see how many of the risk factors you have; these are the risk factors that affect your LDL goal.

__**Cigarette smoking**

__**High blood pressure** (140/90 mmHg or higher or you are taking blood pressure medication)

__**Low HDL cholesterol** (less than 40 mg/dL)*

__**Family history of early heart disease** (heart disease in father or brother before age 55; heart disease in mother or sister before age 65)

__**Age** (men 45 years or older; women 55 years or older)

Total number of risk factors from the list: ______

Step 2: How many major risk factors do you have? (If your HDL cholesterol is 60 mg/dL or higher, subtract 1 from your total count. If you have 2 or more risk factors on the list, use the online Framingham scoring tables (which include your cholesterol levels) to find your risk score. Risk score refers to the chance of having a heart attack in the next 10 years, given as a percentage.

From the National Cholesterol Education Program:

`http://hp2010.nhlbihin.net/atpiii/calculator.asp`

My risk score is ________%.

Step 3: Use your medical history, number of risk factors, and risk score to find your risk of developing heart disease or having a heart attack in the table below.

Risk of Developing Heart Disease or Having a Heart Attack

If You Have	You Are in Category
Heart disease, diabetes, or risk score more than 20%*	I. High Risk
2 or more risk factors and risk score 10 – 20%	II. Next Highest Risk
2 or more risk factors and risk score less than 10%	III. Moderate Risk
0 or 1 risk factor	IV. Low-to-Moderate Risk

* Means that more than 20 of 100 people in this category will have a heart attack within 10 years.

My risk category is ________________________.

Even though obesity and physical inactivity are not counted in this list, they can easily lead to health problems and you should consider how they contribute positively or negatively to your risk factors on the above table.

My weight __ positively __negatively affects my risk factors.
My activity level __ positively __negatively affects my risk factors.

Both weight loss and activity level are two things that you have control over and each of them is important when you are trying to reduce your risk of heart disease or heart attack.

Treating High Cholesterol

The main goal of cholesterol-lowering treatment is to lower your LDL level enough to reduce your risk of developing heart disease or having a heart attack. The higher your risk, the lower your LDL goal number will be. There are two main ways to lower your cholesterol:

1. Weight Management. Losing weight if you are overweight can help lower LDL. It is especially important for those with a cluster of risk factors that includes high triglyceride and/or low HDL levels, and being overweight with a large waist measurement (more than 40 inches for men and more than 35 inches for women).

2. Physical Activity. Regular physical activity (30 minutes on most, if not all, days) is recommended for everyone (with, of course, doctor's approval). It can help raise your HDL and lower your LDL and is especially important for those with high triglyceride and/or low HDL levels who are overweight and have a large waist measurement.

Recommended Foods. Foods low in saturated fat include fat-free or 1 percent dairy products, lean meats, fish, skinless poultry, whole grain foods, and fruits and vegetables.

Look for soft margarines (liquid or tub varieties) that are low in saturated fat and contain little or no trans fat (another type of dietary fat that can raise your cholesterol level).

Limit foods high in cholesterol such as liver and other organ meats, egg yolks, and full-fat dairy products.

Good sources of soluble fiber include oats, certain fruits (such as oranges and pears), vegetables (such as brussels sprouts and carrots), and dried peas and beans.

Drug Treatment

Always consult with your doctor before beginning any dietary or activity changes. If your cholesterol is high and your doctor recommends drug treatment, you will still need to make lifestyle changes. This will keep the dose of medicine as low as possible, and lower your risk in other ways as well. includes losing weight if needed, increasing physical activity, and quitting smoking.

Fat: The Good and the Bad

Fat is a major source of energy and aids your body in absorbing vitamins. It's important for proper growth, development and keeping you healthy. Fat provides taste to foods and helps you feel full. Fats are an especially important source of calories and nutrients for infants and toddlers. Dietary fat also plays a major role in your cholesterol levels.

But, as you've seen, not all fats are the same. You should try to avoid:

- **Saturated fats** such as butter, solid shortening, lard and fatback.
- **Trans fats,** found in vegetable shortenings, some margarines, crackers, cookies, snack foods and other foods made with or fried in partially hydrogenated oils.

Try to replace these fats with oils such as corn, canola, olive, safflower, soybean and sunflower. Of course, eating too much of any kind of fat, even healthy fat, will put on extra weight.

Nutrition Facts Labels

In Chapter 4 you looked at the Nutrition Facts labels to see the sodium content in packaged food. You can also find information about saturated fat, trans fat and cholesterol on these labels. You can even see how many calories come from each kind of fat. (The Nutrition Facts calorie information is a useful reminder that "non-fat" doesn't necessarily mean "dietetic" or low calorie.)

Fat Information on the Nutrition Facts Label

Phrase	What it Means
Fat-free	Less than 0.5 g per serving
Low saturated fat	1 g or less per serving and 15% or less of calories from saturated fat
Low-fat	3 g or less per serving
Reduced fat	At least 25 percent less fat than the regular version
Light in fat	Half the fat compared to the regular version

Nutrition Facts

Cheese Sauce
Serving Size 1/2 cup (130g)
Servings Per Container 2

Amount Per Serving ½ cup	
Calories 250	Calories from Fat 150
	% Daily Value*
Total Fat 14 g	**22%**
Saturated Fat 9g	**45%**
***Trans* Fat** 0g	**0%**
Cholesterol 55mg	**18%**
Sodium 150mg	**6%**
Potassium 270mg	**8%**
Total Carbohydrate 5g	**2%**
Dietary Fiber 1g	**4%**
Sugar 3g	
Protein 1g	
Vitamin A 5%	**Vitamin C** 30%
Calcium 4%	**Iron** 4%

The label above shows that a half a cup of this cheese sauce has 22% of the total Daily Value (DV) for fat. Of that 14 grams, 9 grams—45%—is saturated fat. It has no transfat, but has 18% of the DV of cholesterol.

Half a cup of this cheese sauce gives you 250 calories, and more than half of those calories are from fat. This is obviously a poor food choice as it has large quantities of calories and saturated fat and few nutrients.

The American Heart Association's Nutrition Committee recommends that Americans consume less than 25-36% of their daily calories from fat, preferably less, and less than 7% of that from saturated fat.

They recommend limiting cholesterol to "less than 300 mg per day, for most people. If you have coronary heart disease or your LDL cholesterol level is 100 mg/dL or greater, limit your cholesterol intake to less than 200 milligrams a day." You can read more about their recommendations on the American Heart Association website: `http://www.heart.org`

Reminder

Saturated Fat. Eating too much saturated fat, the type of fat that is solid at room temperature, may increase risk of heart disease.

Trans Fat. Eating too much *trans* fat, which is made when liquid vegetable oil is processed to become solid, also may increase risk of heart disease.

Cholesterol. Eating too much cholesterol a fatty substance found only in animal-based products, may clog arteries and lead to heart disease.

Try to consume less than 25-36% of your daily calories from fat—preferably even less than that—and less than 7% from saturated fat.

NIH has the Following Tips for Limiting "Bad" Fats:

- Trim extra fat and skin on meats and poultry before cooking.
- Instead of frying, try baking, steaming, grilling or broiling.
- Use olive or canola oil instead of butter or margarine.
- Choose margarines with liquid vegetable oil listed as the first ingredient.
- Look for recipes that use applesauce instead of butter or oil.
- Instead of making a double-crust pie, try a single crust.
- Serve fruits for dessert.
- Use fat-free or low-fat dairy products when possible.
- Avoid cream dips, gravy and whipped cream.
- Use broth-based sauces, vinegar, lemon and herbs to add flavor, not fat.

An NIH tip I will use from the list above is to: ________________

____

____

Something I want to remember from this chapter is: __________

____

____

8

Get Ready, Get Set....

The DASH eating plan ("Dietary Approaches to Stop Hypertension") is an easy-to-follow, heart-healthy diet that will help you lose weight, reduce the risk factors for many diseases including diabetes and heart disease, and also help prevent or reduce high blood pressure.

This diet is low in sodium, cholesterol, saturated and total fat, and high in fruits and vegetables, fiber, potassium, and low-fat dairy products. These are all recommended healthy lifestyle choices, and it is no surprise that U.S. News and World Report chose DASH as the #1 Best Diet for Healthy Eating as well as the #1 Best Overall Diet. (You can read more about their conclusions at *U.S. News and World Report* online: `http://health.usnews.com/best-diet`.

Making other lifestyle changes while on DASH—especially getting more physical activity—will, of course, give you the biggest benefits.

4 Different Calorie Plans

DASH has several eating plans for different calorie requirements, and centers around daily servings from various food groups. The chart on page 65 shows the number of different food servings on a DASH plan of 2,000 calories per day. The number of servings you require will depend on your individual calorie needs, but it is easy to tweak any plan to meet your personal goal. Just add or subtract a glass of milk, an extra slice of bread or a serving of fruit, based on calories. Because you are encouraged to choose fresh, natural foods over processed ones, adjusting the plan by adding or removing a daily serving from any food group is easy to do. The charts in Chapter 9 give the DASH daily food group/servings plans at four different calorie counts.

Dieting is not only a physical activity; it also makes mental and emotional demands on you. You are more likely to stay on a diet if you are aware of what happened in the past that led to you to gain weight. It is also helpful to recognize your past patterns and current habits—where and when you are most likely to break your diet, the reasons that you eat other than hunger, how often you exercise—and other actions and feelings that will affect your dieting success. To help you understand these better before you begin DASH, this chapter includes two copies of the journal pages. These are for you to keep a record of your current eating and exercise habits for the next two days. From looking at your current patterns before beginning DASH, you will be able to anticipate some of the likely difficulties—and then plan ahead for success.

Record Your Current Food Choices for 2 Days

Fill in the "What Did I Eat and How Much Did I Exercise?" chart on the next page. Compare what you usually eat with the servings on the DASH plan—and also make a note of your activity level. These are the same journal forms you will be using to track your DASH diet progress later in your *60 Day DASH Weight Loss and Fitness Journal*. But, for now, you are only using the journal pages to record everything you eat or drink in the next two days. Also record the exercise you do. Don't change any habits—this is just for you to see the strengths and weaknesses of your current lifestyle choices.

Compare Your Habits with DASH

After you complete two days of your journal, you will compare your current eating patterns with the healthy servings allowed on DASH. This way you can see your current food choices and will better understand how your habits and decisions have lead to weight gain. This comparison will also help you decide what changes you need to make to begin DASH. In changing your eating habits with DASH, remember to pay particular attention to reducing salt, fats, and processed foods.

What Did I Eat and How Much Did I Exercise?

List what you eat and drink each day. Also include your activity level.

DAY 1 **Date: _______________**

Time	Food	Notes

DAY 2 Date: ______________

Time	Food	Notes*

For Day 1:

Did you get 6-8 8 oz. glasses of water a day? ___Yes ___No

Did you usually exercise? □ Yes □ No _________ minutes/day.

My exercise/activity was:_________________________________

For Day 2:

Did you get 6-8 8 oz. glasses of water a day? ___Yes ___No

Did you usually exercise? □ Yes □ No _________ minutes/day.

My exercise/activity was:_________________________________

Here is a look at the DASH Diet food groups and servings for 2000 calories.

The Daily DASH Diet

2000 Calorie Plan (reduce or add food as needed)

Sodium Goal: 2300 mg/day or 1500 mg/day

Grains – 4-6 servings per day; try for whole grains

□ □ □ □ □ □

Vegetables – 4-6 servings per day; (serving = ½ c)

□ □ □ □ □ □

Fruit – 4-6 servings per day; (serving= ½ c.)

□ □ □ □ □ □

Milk & Milk Products – 2-3 servings (serving = 8oz)

□ □ □

Meat, Chicken, Fish – 6 servings (1 serving =1oz)

□ □ □ □ □ □

Nuts, seeds, and legumes — 4–5 per week

□ □ □ □ □ □

Fats and oils – 2-3 per day

□ □ □

Sweets and sugar – 5 servings or less per week

□ □ □ □ □

How did you do? Look below for a Self Assessment Questionnaire that will help you see which parts of DASH you need to concentrate on.

Self-Assessment Questions

After you've documented your current eating habits, you're ready to begin DASH.. The following questions will help.

	√ Yes	No
My typical diet compared with the DASH Diet:		
1. **Fiber.** I need to add #___ daily servings of fiber .	☐	☐
2. **Vegetables.** I need to add ___ servings of vegetables.	☐	☐
3. **Fruit.** I need to add ___daily servings of fruit.	☐	☐
4. **Milk.** I need to add ___servings of milk products .	☐	☐
5. **Protein.** I need to add ___servings of meat/fish/poultry.	☐	☐
6. **Fats.** I have the amount (and kinds) of oils and fats.	☐	☐
7. **Sweets.** I stay within the amount of sugar and sweets.	☐	☐

8. **Weaknesses.** I know that I am more likely to overeat when I . . . .

____

9. **Strengths.** What is the best thing about your current eating habits? (for example, eating regular meals, liking vegetables and fruit, getting milk or fiber, avoiding sweets in drinks, etc.)

____

____

10. **Exercise.** Do you exercise every day now? __Yes __No

What is your plan for adding (more) exercise to your day?

____

____

____

Now think about how you choose the food you eat throughout a typical day. Then answer this question: "What is one habit about how I choose food that I will change starting right now?" Write that, and any other thoughts about your dietary problems, past and present, and possible solutions in the space below. Be sure to include any specific changes you want to make. Also, you can write down any healthy habits you currently have, the DASH foods you like, activities you do regularly, anything good about your overall health, including your blood pressure and cholesterol.

This is a good time to think about what you've read so far and to express your feelings about change. Why do you want to lose weight? What changes do you need to make to diet and lifestyle choices? It is also good to think about your weaknesses—and strengths—when it comes to diet and exercise. When and how will you begin? What is your plan to stay motivated, since we know there are always so many temptations—and times when diets become difficult to stay on? There is also space below to write down anything that you want to remember from previous chapters. Most people will not want to write about all of these things, but choose something that you feel is important.

9

The DASH Diet Begins

In Chapter 8 you looked at your current habits and compared them with the DASH eating plan. Again, here is a DASH daily servings plan.

DASH Servings for a 2000 Calorie Plan

Food Groups	Daily Servings	Serving Size
Grains*	6–8	1 slice bread 1 oz dry cereal† 1/2 cup cooked rice, pasta,
Vegetables	4–5	1 cup raw leafy vegetable 1/2 cup chopped raw or cooked 1/2 cup vegetable juice
Fruits	4–5	1 medium fruit 1/4 cup dried fruit 1/2 cup fresh, frozen, or canned 1/2 cup fruit juice
Fat-free or low-fat milk products	2–3	1 cup milk or yogurt 1 ½ oz cheese
Lean meats, poultry, and fish	6 or less	1 oz cooked meat, poultry, fish 1 egg‡
Nuts, seeds, and legumes	4–5 per week	1/3 cup or 1 ½ oz nuts 2 Tbsp peanut butter 1/2 cup cooked dry beans; peas
Fats and oils§	2–3	1 tsp soft margarine. oil 1 Tbsp mayonnaise 2 Tbsp salad dressing
Sweets and Sugar	5 or less/week	1 Tbsp sugar or jelly or jam

The DASH Diet Plan

DASH encourages you to reduce or eliminate processed food and to count servings from each food group. When you begin the DASH Diet, your diet journal will make it easy for you to keep track of the food groups every day.

Checking off each food group and serving every day in your journal will make it easy to see that you are staying with your diet. It gives you a visual reminder of your daily progress. (Also, it makes it harder to cheat if you resolve to "not eat anything not on DASH until all my food group servings have been met today." Chances are that if you do this, you will not be hungry and also not reach impulsively throughout the day for foods that are not on DASH.

Slow, Steady Weight Loss

People who need to lose weight should aim for slow, steady weight loss by eating less and moving more.

For overweight or obese adults, it's beneficial to lose even a small amount of weight, and it is especially important not to gain more weight. If you need to lose weight, see if you can cut 500 calories each day from sugar, unhealthy fats, and alcohol. These small cuts will, over time, lead to great benefits.

In Chapter 4 you discovered how many calories you need to have each day based on your height, weight goal and your activity level. For your convenience, we've included this chart on the next page so that you can refer to it when choosing your DASH Diet Plan on the pages that follow.

My usual activity level is

__sedentary __moderately active __active

My daily calories should be: ____________________

How Many Calories Do You Need?
Based on Gender, Age, and Activity Level

Gender	Age/Yrs.	Calories		
		Sedentary	**Moderately Active**	**Active**
Child	2 - 3	1,000	1,000 - 1,400	1,000 - 1,400
Female	4 - 8	1,200	1,400 - 1,600	1,400 - 1,800
	9 - 13	1,600	1,600 - 2,000	1,800 - 2,200
	14 - 18	1,800	2,000	2,400
	19 - 30	2,000	2,000 - 2,200	2,400
	31 - 50	1,800	2,000	2,400
	51+	1,600	1,800	2,000 - 2,200
Male	4 - 8	1,400	1,400 - 1,600	1,600 - 2,000
	9 - 13	1,800	1,800 - 2,200	2,000 - 2,600
	14 - 18	2,200	2,400 - 2,800	2,800 - 3,200
	19 - 30	2,400	2,600 - 2,800	3,000
	31 - 50	2,200	2,400 - 2,600	2,800 - 3,000
	51+	2,000	2,200 - 2,400	2,400 - 2,800

Calorie Ranges. The calorie ranges shown are to accommodate needs of different ages within the group. For adults, fewer calories are needed at older ages. For more information on the *Dietary Guidelines for Americans*, go online to: **www.healthierus.gov/dietaryguidelines.**

These levels are based on Estimated Energy Requirements (EER) from the Institute of Medicine (IOM) Dietary Reference Intakes macro-nutrients report,2002, calculated by gender, age, and activity level for reference-sized individuals. "Reference size," as determined by IOM, is based on median height and weightfor ages up to age 18 years of age and median height and weight for that height to give a Body Mass Index(BMI) of 21.5 for adult females and 22.5 for adult males.

Now look at the DASH Diet Plans on the following pages and choose the one that's closest to your calorie needs. (Remember, it is easy to adjust a calorie count by adding or subtracting daily servings of lean protein, grain or dairy.)

The Daily DASH Diet

__1600 Calorie Plan

The Daily DASH Diet
1600 calories

Food Groups	Servings
Grains*	6
Vegetables	3 - 4
Fruits	4
Milk and milk products, fat-free or lowfat	**2 - 3**
Lean meats, poultry, and fish	3 - 6
Nuts, seeds, and legumes	3/week
Fats and oils	2
Sweets and added sugars	0

*Whole grains are recommended for most grain servings as a good source of fiber and nutrients.

The Daily DASH Diet

__2000 Calorie Plan

The Daily DASH Diet
2000 calories

Food Groups	Servings
Grains*	6 - 8
Vegetables	4 - 5
Fruits	4 - 5
Milk and milk products, fat-free or lowfat	2 - 3
Lean meats, poultry, and fish	6 or less
Nuts, seeds, and legumes	4 - 5/week
Fats and oils	2 - 3
Sweets and added sugars	≤2

*Whole grains are recommended for most grain servings as a good source of fiber and nutrients.

The Daily DASH Diet
__2600 Calorie Plan

The Daily DASH Diet
2600 calories

Food Groups	Servings
Grains*	10 - 11
Vegetables	5 - 6
Fruits	5 - 6
Milk and milk products, fat-free or lowfat	3
Lean meats, poultry, and fish	6
Nuts, seeds, and legumes	1
Fats and oils	2 - 3
Sweets and added sugars	3

*Whole grains are recommended for most grain servings as a good source of fiber and nutrients.

The Daily DASH Diet
__3100 Calorie Plan

The Daily DASH Diet
3100 calories

Food Groups	Servings
Grains*	12 - 13
Vegetables	6
Fruits	6
Milk and milk products, fat-free or lowfat	3 - 4
Lean meats, poultry, and fish	6 - 9
Nuts, seeds, and legumes	1
Fats and oils	2 - 3
Sweets and added sugars	4

*Whole grains are recommended for most grain servings as a good source of fiber and nutrients.

Below is an example of a typical DASH eating plan. You can use this to work out a plan based food you like. The next chapter gives you DASH menus for a week, along with easy to follow low-salt recipes.

DASH: A Sample Diet

A Day with the DASH Eating Plan for a 2000 Calorie Plan

Breakfast
oatmeal, 1/2 cup instant
bagel, 1 mini whole wheat:
peanut butter, 1 Tbsp
banana, 1 medium
milk, 1 cup low-fat

Lunch
chicken breast sandwich
    chicken breast, 2 slices (3 oz) skinless
    bread, 2 slices whole wheat
    cheddar cheese, reduced-fat, 1 slice (3/4 oz) natural
    lettuce, 1 large leaf romaine
    tomato, 2 slices
    mayonnaise, 1 Tbsp, low-fat
cantaloupe 1 cup chunks
apple juice 1 cup

Dinner
spaghetti, 1 cup cooked
spaghetti sauce, 3/4 cup low-salt vegetarian
Parmesan cheese, 3 Tbsp
Spinach salad:
    spinach leaves, 1 cup fresh
    carrots, 1/4 cup fresh grated
    mushrooms, 1/4 cup fresh sliced
    vinegar and oil dressing, 1 Tbsp
corn, 1/2 cup cooked from frozen
pears, 1/2 cup canned juice pack

Snacks
almonds, 1/3 cup unsalted
apricots, 1/4 cup dried
yogurt, 1 cup fruit fat-free, no sugar added

Tips on Eating the DASH Way

Start small. Make gradual changes in your eating habits.

Center your meal around carbohydrates, such as pasta, rice, beans, or vegetables.

Treat meat as one part of the whole meal, instead of the focus.

Use fruits or low fat, low-calorie foods such as sugar free gelatin for desserts and snacks.

DASH emphasizes whole grains, fruits and vegetables. Read below for some ways that you can make good choices with each of these food groups.

Fiber and Whole Grains

Whole grains are recommended for most grain servings as a good source of fiber and nutrients. Serving sizes vary between ½ cup and 1¼ cups, depending on the cereal type. You can check the product's Nutrition Facts label for information about fiber.

Fiber, particularly from whole grain foods, is very important on DASH. Each of the fiber servings below is equivalent to 3 ounces of whole grains.

Fiber Equivalents (All equal 3 oz. of whole grain)

- **One slice (1 ounce) of whole-grain bread,**
- **1/2 cup brown rice**
- **1/2 cup of oatmeal**

Many packaged foods have fiber information on the front of the package. For example, the package might say "excellent source of fiber," "rich in fiber," or "high in fiber." The Nutrition Facts label will list the amount of dietary fiber in a serving and the % Daily Value (% DV).

Fiber % Daily Value (DV) on Label

Look at the % DV column on the Nutrition Facts label.

Low. 5% DV or less is low in dietary fiber.
High. 20% DV or more is high.

Whole Grain Foods: Look at the Product Labels

For many, but not all, "whole-grain" food products, the words "whole" or "whole grain" may appear before the name (e.g., whole-wheat bread). But, because whole-grain foods cannot necessarily be identified by their color or name (brown bread, 9-grain bread, hearty grains bread, mixed grain bread, etc. are not always "whole-grain"), you need to look at the ingredient list.

The whole grain should be the first ingredient listed.

"Whole Grains" with Many Names

The following are some examples of different kinds of whole grain products:

- whole wheat
- brown rice
- quinoa
- buckwheat
- whole oats/oatmeal whole rye
- bulgur (cracked wheat) sorghum
- whole grain barley
- popcorn millet
- wild rice triticale

**Make at least half your grains whole grains.
Eat at least 3 ounces of them daily.**

The DASH eating plan has more daily servings of fruits, vegetables, and whole grain foods than you may be used to eating. Because the plan is high in fiber, it can cause bloating and diarrhea in some people. To avoid these problems, increase your intake of fruit, vegetables, and whole grain foods gradually.

Choosing Fruits and Vegetables

Make most of your fruit and vegetable choices fresh, frozen, canned, or dried, rather than fruit juice.

Vitamin C

• **Fruits --** oranges, kiwi, strawberries, guava, papaya, and cantaloupe.

• **Vegetables.** Good choices include: broccoli, peppers, tomatoes, cabbage (especially Chinese cabbage), brussels sprouts, and potatoes. Leafy greens such as romaine lettuce, turnip greens, and spinach are also nutritious.

Vitamin A (carotenoids)

• **Fruits** -- **Orange fruits** like mango, cantaloupe, apricots, and red or pink grapefruit.

• **Vegetables** -- **Green and orange**. Eat more dark green veggies such as broccoli, kale, and other dark leafy greens. Try orange veggies, such as carrots, sweet potatoes, pumpkin, and winter squash.

Bright orange vegetables like carrots, sweet potatoes, and pumpkin.

Tomatoes and tomato products (sauce, paste, and puree), and red sweet pepper.

Leafy greens such as spinach, collards, turnip greens, kale, beet and mustard greens, green leaf lettuce, and romaine lettuce

Remember

If you are unsure what fruit or vegetable to get, think "orange" and "deep green and leafy".

Good DASH Foods to Choose From

Some examples of DASH food possibilities	Nutrition Benefits
Fiber. Whole wheat bread and rolls, whole wheat pasta, English muffin, pita bread, bagel, cereals, grits, oatmeal, brown rice, unsalted pretzels and popcorn	**energy and fiber**
Vegetables. Broccoli, carrots, collards, green beans, green peas, kale, lima beans, potatoes, spinach, squash, sweet potatoes, tomatoes	**potassium, fiber and magnesium**
Fruit. Apples, apricots, bananas, dates, grapes, oranges, grapefruit, grapefruit juice, mangoes, melons, peaches, pineapples, raisins, strawberries, tangerines	**fiber, magnesium, and potassium**
Dairy. Fat-free (skim) or low-fat (1%) milk or buttermilk,fat-free, low-fat, or reduced-fat cheese,fat-free or low-fat regular or frozen yogurt	**calcium and protein**
Protein. Select only lean; trim away visible fats; broil, roast, or poach; remove skin from poultry	**protein and magnesium**
Nuts, beans, seeds. Almonds, hazelnuts, mixed nuts, peanuts, walnuts, sunflower seeds, peanut butter kidney beans, lentils, split peas	**magnesium and energy, ,protein fiber**

Fat. Soft margarine, vegetable oil (including canola, corn, olive, or safflower), low-fat mayonnaise, or light salad dressing

Sweets. Fruit-flavored gelatin, fruit punch, hard candy, jelly, maple syrup, sorbet and ices, sugar

Begin DASH at 2,000 milligrams of sodium

Because it is rich in fruits and vegetables, which are naturally lower in sodium than many other foods, the DASH eating plan makes it easier to consume less salt and sodium. Still, you may want to begin by adopting the DASH eating plan at the level of 2,300 milligrams of sodium per day and then further lower your sodium intake to 1,500 milligrams per day.

Reduce Salt to 2300 mg or 1500 mg of sodium a day
Include Potassium at 4,700 mg of potassium a day

The DASH eating plan emphasizes getting potassium from food, especially fruits and vegetables, to help keep blood pressure levels healthy. A potassium-rich diet may help to reduce elevated or high blood pressure, but be sure to get your potassium from food sources, not from supplements. Many fruits and vegetables, some milk products, and fish are rich sources of potassium.

In general, aim for.....

- 2,300 mg of sodium (or less) per day for adults (1 tsp)
- 1,500 mg of sodium (or less) per day for at-risk adults (⅔ tsp)
- 4,700 mg/day potassium, eaten in food.

Combining the DASH eating plan with a regular physical activity program, such as walking or swimming, will help you lose weight and look better. You can do an activity for 30 minutes at one time, or choose shorter periods of at least 10 minutes each. The important thing is to total about 30 minutes of activity each day. Chapter 11 gives you a variety of ways to do this. But first, let's begin with DASH.

My DASH Plan: Food Preferences and Notes

10

Menus and Recipes

A Week With the DASH Eating Plan

Here is a week of menus from the DASH eating plan. The menus allow you to have a daily sodium level of either 2,300 mg or, by making the noted changes, meals with 1,500 mg. of sodium (some a little more or less, as noted). You'll also find that the menus sometimes call for you to use lower sodium, low-fat, fat-free, or reduced fat versions of products.

The menus are based on 2,000 calories a day—serving sizes should be increased or decreased for other calorie levels. To ease the calculations, some of the serving sizes have been rounded off. Also, some items may be in too small a quantity to have a listed food group serving. Recipes for starred items are given on the later pages. Some of these recipes give changes that can be used to lower their sodium level. Use the changes if you want to follow the DASH eating plan at 1,500 milligrams of sodium per day.

Abbreviations:
oz = ounce
tsp = teaspoon
Tbsp = tablespoon
g = gram
mg = milligram

Day 1 Menu
2300 mg. Sodium*

Breakfast	**Sodium** (mg)
bran flakes cereal, 3/4 cup	220
banana, 1 medium	1
low-fat milk, 1 cup	107
whole wheat bread, 1 slice	149
margarine, 1 tsp soft (tub)*	26
orange juice 1 cup	5
Lunch	
chicken salad*, ¾ cup	179
whole wheat bread, 2 slices	299
Dijon mustard, 1 Tbsp*	373
Salad:	
cucumber slices, ½ c.	1
tomato wedges, ½ c.	5
sunflower seeds, 1Tbsp.	0
Italian dressing, low cal, 1 tsp.	43
fruit cocktail, juice pack, ½ c. j	5
Dinner	
beef, eye of the round, 3 oz.	35
beef gravy, fat free, 2 tsp.	165
green beans, 1 c, sauteed with:	12
½ tsp. canola oil	
baked potato, 1 small	
sour cream, fat-free, 1 Tbsp	
cheddar cheese, grated natural, 1 Tbsp	67
whole wheat roll, 1 small	148
margarine, soft (tub), 1 tsp.	26
apple, 1 small	1
low-fat milk, 1 cup	107
almonds, 1/3 cup	
raisins, ¼ cup	
fruit yogurt, fat-free, no added sugar, ½ cup	86
Total	**2101**

Day 1 - Nutrition Information

Number of Servings by Food Group

Sodium:	2100
Grain	5
Vegetables	5
Fruit	6
Milk Products	2 ½
Meat, fish & poultry	6
Nuts, seeds & legumes	1 ½
Fats and oils	3 ½
Sweets and added sugars	0

Day 1 Menu: To reduce the day's total sodium from 2101 mg sodium to 1507 mg, sodium, make these changes:

Breakfast:

Instead of this	Sodium	**Use this**	Sodium
bran flakes cereal, 3/4 cup	220	shredded wheat cereal (3/4 c)	1
margarine, regular soft (tub)	26	margarine, unsalted soft (tub)	0

Lunch

Chicken salad – remove the salt from the recipe

Instead of this		**Use this**	
mustard, 1 Tbsp Dijon	373	mustard, 1 Tbsp regular	175

Dinner

Instead of this		**Use this**	
cheddar cheese, reduced fat	67	same cheese, but "low sodium"	1

Day 2 Menu
2300 mg. Sodium

Breakfast	**Sodium (mg)**
instant oatmeal, ½ cup*	54
whole wheat bagel, 1 mini	84
peanut butter, 1 Tbsp	81
banana, 1 medium	1
low-fat milk, 1 cup	107
Lunch	
chicken breast sandwich	
chicken breast, skinless 3oz.	65
whole wheat bread, 2 slices	299
cheddar cheese, 1 slice (3/4 oz) reduced fat*	202
romaine lettuce, 1 large leaf	1
tomato, 2 slices	2
mayonnaise, low-fat, 1 Tbsp.	101
cantaloupe chunks, 1 cup	26
apple juice, 1 cup	21
Dinner	
spaghetti, 1 cup	
spaghetti sauce vegetarian, ¾ cup**	479
Parmesan cheese, 3 Tbsp	287
Spinach salad:	
spinach leaves, 1 cup fresh	24
carrots, grated, ¼ cup fresh	19
mushrooms, fresh, sliced, ¼ cup	1
vinaigrette*, 1 Tbsp	1
corn, cooked from frozen, ½ cup	1
pears, canned, juice pack, ½ cup	5
Snacks	
almonds, unsalted 1/3 cup	0
apricots, dried, ¼ cup	3
yogurt, fruit, no sugar added, fat-free, 1 cup	173
Total	**2035**

Day 2 - Number of Servings by Food Group

Sodium:	2,035
Grain	6
Vegetables	5¼
Fruit	7
Milk Products	3
Meat, fish & poultry	3
Nuts, seeds & legumes	1½
Fats and oils	1½
Sweets and added sugars	0

Day 2 Menu: To Reduce from 2035 mg to 1560 mg Sodium

Breakfast

Instead of this	Sodium	**Use this**	Sodium
instant oatmeal, ½ cup*	54	regular oatmeal 1/2 cup with1 tsp cinnamon	5

Lunch

Instead of this	Sodium	**Use this**	Sodium
Swiss cheese, 1 slice (3/4 oz) natural, reduced fat,	202	same cheese, low sodium	3

Dinner

Instead of this	Sodium	**Use this**	Sodium
vegetarian spaghetti sauce*	473	use tomato paste (6 oz) low sodium	253

Day 3 Menu

2300 mg. Sodium

Breakfast	**Sodium** (mg)
bran flakes cereal (¾ cup)	220
banana, 1 medium	1
low-fat milk, 1 cup	107
whole wheat bread, 1 slice	146
margarine, 1 tsp. soft (tub)	26
orange juice, 1 cup	6
Lunch	
beef barbecue sandwich	
beef, eye of round, 2 oz.	26
cheddar cheese, reduced fat, 2 slices (1½ oz)	409
barbecue sauce, 1 tsp.	156
hamburger bun, 1	183
romaine lettuce, 1 leaf	1
tomato slices, 2	2
potato salad, 1 cup new*	17
orange, 1 medium	0
Dinner	
cod, 3 oz.	70
lemon juice, 1 tsp	1
brown rice, ½ cup	5
spinach, cooked from frozen	184
sauteed with canola oil, 1 tsp.	0
almonds, 1 Tbsp., slivered	
cornbread muffin, 1 small (with oil)	119
margarine, 1 tsp. soft (tub)	26
Snacks	
fruit yogurt, fat-free, 1 cup (no added sugar)	173
sunflower seeds, unsalted, 1 Tbsp	0
graham cracker rectangles, 2 large	156
peanut butter, 1 Tbsp.	81
Total	**2114**

Number of Servings by Food Group

Grain	7
Vegetables	4 ¾
Fruit	4
Milk Products	3
Meat, fish & poultry	5
Nuts, seeds & legumes	1 ¼
Fats and oils	3
Sweets and added sugars	0

Day 3 Menu: To Reduce from 2114 mg to 1447 mg Sodium

Breakfast:

Instead of this	Sodium	**Use this**	Sodium
bran flakes cereal, ¾ cup	220	2 cups puffed wheat cereal	1
margarine, regular soft (tub)	26	margarine, unsalted soft (tub)	0

Lunch

cheddar cheese, 2 slices (1½ oz) reduced fat	405	cheddar cheese, 2 slices (1½ oz) reduced fat, low sodium	9

Dinner

margarine, regular soft (tub)	26	margarine, unsalted soft (tub)	0

Day 4 Menu

2300 mg. Sodium

Breakfast	**Sodium (mg)**
whole wheat bread, 1 slice	149
margarine, soft (tub), 1 tsp	26*
yogurt, fat-free, fruit no added sugar	173
peach, 1 medium	0
grape juice, ½ cup	4
Lunch	
ham and cheese sandwich:	
ham, low-fat, low salt, 2 oz*	549
cheddar cheese, natural, reduced fat, 1 slice (3/4 oz)	202
whole wheat bread, 2 slices	299
romaine lettuce, 1 large leaf	1
tomato, 2 slices	2
mayonnaise, low-fat, 1 Tbsp	101
carrot sticks, 1 cup	84
Dinner	
chicken and Spanish rice (recipe) *	341
green peas, 1 cup, sauteed iwth	115
canola oil, 1 tsp.	0
cantaloupe chunks, 1 cup	26
low-fat milk, 1 cup	107
Snacks	
almonds, unsalted, 1/3 cup	0
apple juice, 1 cup	21
apricots ¼ cup	3
low-fat milk, 1 cup	107
Total	**2312**

Day Four Food Group Servings:

Grain	4
Vegetables	4 ¾
Fruit	7
Milk Products	3½
Meat, fish & poultry	5
Nuts, seeds & legumes	1
Fats and oils	3
Sweets and added sugars	0

Day 4 Menu: To Reduce from 2312 mg to 1436 mg Sodium

Breakfast

Instead of this	Sodium	Use this	Sodium
margarine, regular soft (tub)	26	margarine, unsalted soft (tub)	0

Lunch

Instead of this	Sodium	Use this	Sodium
2 oz. ham, low-fat, low sodium,	549	2 oz. roast beef tenderloin	23
2 slices (1½ oz) reduced fat	405	cheddar cheese, 2 smlices (1½ oz) reduced fat, low sodium	9

Dinner

Instead of this	Sodium	Use this	Sodium
tomato sauce, 1 can (8 oz).	341	tomato sauce (4 oz) low sodium and 1 4 oz can of regular sauce	241

Day 5 Menu

2300 mg. Sodium

Breakfast	**Sodium (mg)**
whole grain oat rings cereal, 1 cup	273
banana, 1 medium	
low fat milk, 1 cup	
raisin bagel, 1 medium	272
peanut butter, 1 Tbsp	81
orange juice, 1 cup	5

Lunch	
tuna salad plate:	
tuna salad, ½ cup (recipe)	
romaine lettuce, 1 large leaf	1
whole wheat bread, 1 slice	149
cucumber slices, 1 cup fresh	2
tomato wedges, ½ cup	5
vinaigrette dressing, 1 Tbsp	133
cottage cheese, low fat, ½ cup	459
pineapple, canned, juice pack, ½ cup	
almonds, unsalted	0

Dinner	
turkey meatloaf (recipe), 3 oz	205
baked potato, 1 small	14
sour cream, fat free, 1 Tbsp	21
cheddar cheese, reduced fat grated, 1 Tbsp	67
scallion stalk, 1, chopped	1
collard greens, 1 cup, sauteed with	85
canola oil, 1 tsp	
whole wheat roll, 1 small	

Snacks	
peach, 1 medium	0
fruit yogurt, fat free, 1 cup (no added sugar)	173
sunflower seeds, unsalted, 2 Tbsp	0

Day Five Food Group Servings:

Sodium:	2,373
Grain	5
Vegetables	6 ¼
Fruit	5
Milk Products	2 ¼
Meat, fish & poultry	6
Nuts, seeds & legumes	1 ¾
Fats and oils	2
Sweets and added sugars	0

Day 5 Menu: To Reduce from 2373 to 1519 mg Sodium

Breakfast

Instead of	Sodium	**Use this:**	Sodium
oat rings cereal, 1 cup whole grain	273	shredded wheat, 1 cup, frosted	4
peanut butter, 1 Tbsp	81	peanut butter, 1 Tbsp, unsalted	3

Lunch

whole wheat bread, 1 slice	149	whole wheat crackers, 6 low sodium	
vinaigrette dressing 1 Tbsp	133	yogurt dressing, 2 Tbsp fat-free†	66

Dinner

turkey meatloaf recipe	205	substitute low-sodium ketchup	74
cheddar cheese, 1 Tbsp reduced fat, grated	67	use low-sodium cheddar	1
small whole wheat roll, 1	148	melba toast crackers, 6 small	1
Mustard, Dijon, 1 Tbsp	373	mustard, regular, 1 Tbsp	175

Day 6 Menu

2300 mg. Sodium

Breakfast	**Sodium (mg)**
1 low-fat granola bar	81
1 medium banana	1
1/2 cup fruit yogurt, fat-free, no sugar added	86
1 cup orange juice	5
1 cup low-fat milk	107
Lunch	
turkey breast sandwich:	
turkey breast, 3 oz	48
whole wheat bread, 2 slices	299
romaine lettuce, 1 large leaf	1
tomato, 2 slices	2
mayonnaise, low-fat, 2 tsp	67
mustard, 1 Tbsp Dijon	373
broccoli, 1 cup steamed cooked from frozen	11
orange, 1 medium	0
Dinner	
3 oz spicy baked fish*	50
1 cup scallion rice†	18
spinach sauté:	
1/2 cup spinach, cooked from frozen,	92
sautéed with: 2 tsp canola oil	0
almonds, 1 Tbsp slivered, unsalted	0
carrots, 1 cup cooked from frozen	84
whole wheat roll,1 small	148
margarine, 1 tsp soft (tub)	26
cookie, 1 small	60
Snacks	
peanuts, 2 Tbsp, unsalted	1
milk, 1 cup low-fat	107
apricots, 1/4 cup dried	3
Totals	**1,671**

Day Six Food Group Servings:

Grain	6
Vegetables	5 ¾
Fruit	5
Milk Products	2 ½
Meat, fish & poultry	6
Nuts, seeds & legumes	¾
Fats and oils	3 ⅔
Sweets and added sugars	1

Day 6 Menu: To Reduce from 1671 to 1472 mg Sodium

Lunch

Instead of this:	Sodium	Use this:	Sodium
mustard, Dijon, 1 Tbsp.	373	mustard, regular,	175

Day 7 Menu

2300 mg. Sodium

Breakfast	**Sodium (mg)**
whole grain oat rings, 1 cup	273
banana, 1 medium	1
low -fat milk	107
fruit yogurt, fat-free, no added sugar, 1 cup	173
Lunch	
tuna salad sandwich	
tuna, drained, rinsed, ½ cup	39
mayonnaise, low-fat, 1 Tbsp.	101
romaine lettuce leaf, 1 large	1
tomato, 2 slices	2
whole wheat bread, 2 slices	299
apple, 1 medium	1
low-fat milk, 1 cup	107
Dinner	
zucchini lasagna, 1/6 recipe	368
salad:	
spinach leaves, fresh, 1 cup	24
tomato wedges, 1 cup	9
croutons, seasoned, 2 Tbsp	62
vinaigrette dressing, 1 Tbsp reduced calorie	133
sunflower seeds, 1 Tbsp	0
whole wheat roll, 1 small	148
margarine, soft (tub), 1 tsp	45
grape juice, 1 cup	8
Snacks	
almonds, unsalted, 1/3 cup	0
apricots, dry, 1/4 cup	3
whole wheat crackers, 6	166
Total	**2312**

Day 7 Food Group Servings:

Grain	8 ¼
Vegetables	4 ¾
Fruit	5
Milk Products	4
Meat, fish & poultry	3
Nuts, seeds & legumes	1 ½
Fats and oils	2 ½
Sweets and added sugars	0

Day 7 Menu: To Reduce from 2069 mg to 1500 mg Sodium

Breakfast

Instead of this:	Sodium	Use this:	Sodium
whole grain oat rings, 1 cup	273	oatmeal, regular, 1 cup	5

Lunch

Instead of this:	Sodium	Use this:	Sodium
vinaigrette dressing, 1 Tbsp reduced calorie	133	vinaigrette, low sodium 1 Tbsp(recipe)	1
margarine, soft (tub), 1 tsp	45	margarine, soft, (tub) unsalted, 1 tsp	0

Dinner

zucchini recipe (1/6, 368) substitute cottage cheese, low-fat, 165
no salt added (recipe)

Recipes: Day 1 -7

Day 1 Recipes

Chicken Salad

3 1/4 cups chicken breast, cooked, cubed, and skinless
1/4 cup celery, chopped
1 Tbsp lemon juice
1/2 tsp onion powder
1/8 tsp salt*
3 Tbsp mayonnaise, low-fat

1. Bake chicken, cut into cubes, and refrigerate.
2. In a large bowl combine rest of ingredients, add chilled chicken and mix well.

Sodium: 179 mg per serving
Serving Size: 3/4 cup. 176 calories per serving.

** To reduce sodium, omit the 1/8 tsp of added salt. New sodium content for each serving is 120 mg.*

Day 2 Recipes

Vegetarian Spaghetti Sauce

2 Tbsp olive oil
2 small onions, chopped
3 cloves garlic, chopped
1 1/4 cups zucchini, sliced
1 Tbsp oregano, dried
1 Tbsp basil, dried
1 8 oz can tomato sauce
1 6 oz can tomato paste*
2 medium tomatoes, chopped
1 cup water

Vegetarian Spaghetti Sauce (cont.)

1. In a medium skillet, heat oil. Sauté onions, garlic, and zucchini in oil for 5 minutes on medium heat.
2. Add remaining ingredients and simmer covered for 45 minutes. Serve over spaghetti.

** To reduce sodium, use a 6-oz can of low-sodium tomato paste. New sodium content for each serving is 253 mg.*

Makes 6 servings. Sodium: 479 mg per serving
Serving Size: 3/4 cup. 105 calories per serving.

Vinaigrette Salad Dressing

1 bulb garlic, separated and peeled
1/2 cup water
1 Tbsp red wine vinegar
1/4 tsp honey
1 Tbsp virgin olive oil
1/4 tsp black pepper

1. Place the garlic cloves into a small saucepan and pour enough water (about 1/2 cup) to cover them.
2. Bring water to a boil, then reduce heat and simmer until garlic is tender, about 15 minutes.
3. Reduce the liquid to 2 Tbsp and increase the heat for 3 minutes.
4. Pour the contents into a small sieve over a bowl, and with a wooden spoon, mash the garlic through the sieve into the bowl.
5. Whisk the vinegar into the garlic mixture; incorporate the oil and seasoning.

Serving Size: 2 Tbsp
Sodium: 1 mg per serving. 33 calories per serving.

Day 3 Recipes

New Potato Salad

16 small new potatoes (5 cups)
2 Tbsp olive oil
1/4 cup green onions, chopped
1/4 tsp black pepper
1 tsp dill weed, dried

1. Thoroughly clean potatoes with vegetable brush and water.
2. Boil potatoes for 20 minutes or until tender.
3. Drain and cool potatoes for 20 minutes.
4. Cut potatoes into quarters and mix with olive oil, onions, and spices.
5. Refrigerate until ready to serve.

Makes 5 servings. Sodium: 17 mg per serving.
Serving Size: 1 cup 196 calories per serving.

Day 4 Recipes

Chicken and Spanish Rice

1 cup onions, chopped
3/4 cup green peppers
2 tsp vegetable oil
1 8 oz can tomato sauce
1 tsp parsley, chopped
1/2 tsp black pepper
1 1/4 tsp garlic, minced
5 cups cooked brown rice (cooked in unsalted water)
3 1/2 cups chicken breasts, cooked, skin and bone removed, and diced

Chicken and Spanish Rice (cont.)

1. In a large skillet, sauté onions and green peppers in oil for 5 minutes on medium heat.
2. Add tomato sauce and spices. Heat through.
3. Add cooked rice and chicken. Heat through.

Makes 5 servings. Sodium: 341 mg per servings
Serving Size: 1 ½ cup. 428 calories per serving.

Day 5 Recipes

Turkey Meatloaf

1 pound lean ground turkey
1/2 cup regular oats, dry
1 large egg, whole
1 Tbsp onion, dehydrated flakes
1/4 cup ketchup*

1. Combine all ingredients and mix well.
2. Bake in a loaf pan at 350 °F for 25 minutes or to an internal temperature of 165 °F.
3. Cut into five slices and serve.

Makes 5 servings. Sodium: 205 mg per servings
Serving Size:1 slice (3 oz). 191 calories per serving.

Tuna Salad

2 6 oz cans tuna, water pack
1/2 cup raw celery, chopped
1/3 cup green onions, chopped
61/2 Tbsp mayonnaise, low-fat

Tuna Salad

1. Rinse and drain tuna for 5 minutes. Break apart with a fork.
2. Add celery, onion, and mayonnaise and mix well.

Makes 5 servings. Sodium: 171 mg. per serving.
Serving Size: 1/2 cup 138 calories per serving.

Yogurt Salad Dressing

8 oz plain yogurt, fat-free
1/4 cup mayonnaise, low-fat
2 Tbsp chives, dried
2 Tbsp dill, dried
2 Tbsp lemon juice

1. Mix all ingredients in bowl and refrigerate.

Makes 5 servings . Sodium: 66 mg. per serving
Serving Size: 2 Tbsp 39 calories per serving.

Day 6 Recipes

Spicy Baked Fish

1 pound salmon (or other fish) fillet
1 Tbsp olive oil
1 tsp spicy seasoning, salt-free

1. Preheat oven to 350 °F. Spray a casserole dish with cooking oil spray.
2. Wash and dry fish. Place in dish. Mix oil and seasoning and drizzle over fish.
3. Bake uncovered for 15 minutes or until fish flakes with fork. Cut into 4 pieces. Serve with rice.

Makes 4 servings. Sodium: 50 mg per servings
Serving Size: 1 piece (3 oz) 50 calories per serving

Scallion Rice

4 1/2 cups cooked brown rice (cooked in unsalted water)
1 1/2 tsp bouillon granules, low sodium
1/4 cup scallions (green onions), chopped

1. Cook rice according to directions on the package.
2. Combine the cooked rice, scallions, and bouillon granules and mix well.
3. Measure 1-cup portions and serve.

Makes 5 servings. Sodium: 18 mg per serving
Serving Size: 1 cup   200 calories per serving

Day 7 Recipes

Zucchini Lasagna

1/2 pound cooked lasagna noodles, cooked in unsalted water
3/4 cup part-skim mozzarella cheese, grated
1 1/2 cups cottage cheese,* fat-free
1/4 cup Parmesan cheese, grated
1 1/2 cups raw zucchini, sliced
2 1/2 cups low-sodium tomato sauce
2 tsp basil, dried
2 tsp oregano, dried
1/4 cup onion, chopped
1 clove garlic
1/8 tsp black pepper

1. Preheat oven to 350 °F. Lightly spray a 9- by 13-inch baking dish with vegetable oil spray.
2. In a small bowl, combine 1/8 cup mozzarella and 1 Tbsp Parmesan cheese. Set aside.
3. In a medium bowl, combine remaining mozzarella and Parmesan cheese with all the cottage cheese. Mix well and set aside.

4. Combine tomato sauce with remaining ingredients. Spread a thin layer of tomato sauce in the bottom of the baking dish. Add a third of the noodles in a single layer. Spread half of the cottage cheese mixture on top. Add a layer of zucchini.
5. Repeat layering. Add a thin coating of sauce. Top with noodles, sauce, and reserved cheese mixture. Cover with aluminum foil. 6. Bake 30 to 40 minutes. Cool for 10 to 15 minutes. Cut into 6 portions.

* *To reduce sodium, use low-sodium cottage cheese. New sodium content for each serving is 165 mg*

Makes 6 servings. Sodium: 368 mg per serving
Serving Size: 1 piece 200 calories per serving

11

The Exercise DASH

Exercise is a vital part of any diet plan, and it is especially important to the DASH Diet, with its emphasis on weight loss and improved health and fitness.

Physical Activity and Your Health

If you currently get regular physical activity, congratulations! But if you're not yet getting all the activity you need, you have lots of company. According to the Centers for Disease Control and Prevention (CDC), 60 percent of Americans are not meeting the recommended levels of physical activity. Fully 16 percent of Americans are not active at all. Overall, women tend to be less active than men, and older people are less likely to get regular physical activity than younger individuals.

What does it mean to get "regular physical activity?" To reduce the risk of heart disease, adults need only do about 30 minutes of moderate activity on most days of the week; exercising every day is obviously even better. This level of activity can lower your chances of having a stroke, colon cancer, high blood pressure, diabetes, and other medical problems.

If you're also trying to manage your weight and prevent gradual, unhealthy weight gain, try to get 60 minutes of moderate- to vigorous-intensity activity on most days of the week. At the same time, watch your calories. Take in only enough calories to maintain your weight. Those who are trying to keep weight off should aim a bit higher: try to get 60 to 90 minutes of moderate-intensity activity daily, without taking in extra calories. In the next chapter, you'll find out more about the types of activities that you can easily fit into your routine, as well as ways to break up your activity time into manageable segments.

If you can, aim for at least 30 min of moderate-intensity physical activity on most days of the week. When your heart is beating noticeably faster, the activity is probably moderately intense. Use your *60 Day Weight Loss and Fitness Journal* to record your minutes per day and the activity you chose.

How to Change a Habit of Inactivity

If you're not as active as you should be, take a moment to consider why. Maybe you're just in the habit of traveling by car or bus, even when you're not going far. In your free time, perhaps it's tempting to sit down in front of the TV or computer rather than do something more vigorous. It's easy to get busy—or to feel tired—and decide that it's just simpler to put off that brisk walk or bike ride.

But when you think about the serious problems that physical inactivity can create for your health—and the enormous rewards of getting regular activity—you may want to reconsider.

1. If you're not active now, why do you think that is?

I'm not more active because ________________________________

____

2. What changes could you make in your lifestyle or thinking so that you will become more active?

I would have a more active lifestyle if I didn't ______________________

____

Instead, I will ____

The more you know about the benefits of regular exercise, the more likely you will commit to increasing its importance in your daily routine. Heart disease is the leading causes of death for Americans and your heart is one of the greatest beneficiaries of regular exercise.

The Heart Connection

It is worth repeating: physical inactivity greatly increases your risk of developing heart disease. Heart disease occurs when the arteries that supply blood to the heart muscle become hardened and narrowed, due to a buildup of plaque on the arteries' inner walls. Plaque is the accumulation of fat, cholesterol, and other substances. As plaque continues to build up in the arteries, blood flow to the heart is reduced.

Heart disease can lead to a heart attack. A heart attack happens when a cholesterol-rich plaque bursts and releases its contents into the bloodstream. This causes a blood clot to form over the plaque, totally blocking blood flow through the artery and preventing vital oxygen and nutrients from getting to the heart. A heart attack can cause permanent damage to the heart muscle.

Some people aren't too concerned about heart disease because they think it can be cured with surgery. This is a myth. Heart disease is a life-long condition. It is true that certain procedures can help blood and oxygen flow more easily to the heart. But the arteries remain damaged, which means you are still more likely to have a heart attack. What's more, the condition of your blood vessels will steadily worsen unless you make changes in your daily habits and control other factors that increase risk.

Heart disease is a serious disease—and too often, a fatal one. It is the number one killer of Americans, with 500,000 people in the United States dying of heart disease each year. Many others with heart problems become permanently disabled. That is why it is so vital to take action to prevent this disease. Getting regular physical activity should be part of everyone's heart disease prevention program.

Heart Disease Risk Factors

Risk factors are conditions or habits that make a person more likely to develop a disease. They can also increase the chances that an existing disease will get worse. Certain risk factors for heart disease, such as getting older or having a family history of early heart disease, can't be changed. But physical inactivity is a major risk factor for heart disease that you have control over. You can make a decision to get regular physical activity, and this chapter and the next will help you create a workable, enjoyable program that will help you protect your heart.

Other major risk factors for heart disease that you can change are smoking, high blood pressure, high blood cholesterol, overweight, and diabetes. Every risk factor counts. Research shows that each individual risk factor greatly increases the chances of developing heart disease and having a heart attack. A damaged heart can damage your life, by interfering with enjoyable activities and even keeping you from doing simple things, such as taking a walk or climbing steps.

It is important to know that you have a lot of power to protect your heart health. Getting regular physical activity is an especially important part of your healthy heart program, because physical activity both directly reduces your heart disease risk and it also reduces your chances of developing other risk factors for heart disease. For example, regular physical activity may reduce LDL (bad) cholesterol, increase HDL (good) cholesterol, and lower high blood pressure. It can also protect your heart by helping to prevent and control diabetes. Finally, physical activity can help you lose excess weight or to maintain a desirable weight, which will also help to lower your risk of heart disease.

You Have Control

Physical inactivity is one of several major risk factors for heart disease that you can do something about. The others are:

Smoking. People who smoke are up to six times more likely to suffer a heart attack than nonsmokers, and the risk increases with the number of cigarettes smoked each day. Quitting will greatly reduce your risk. Check with local community groups for free or low-cost programs designed to help people stop smoking.

High Blood Pressure. Also known as hypertension, high blood pressure increases your risk of heart disease, stroke, kidney disease, and congestive heart failure. Your health care provider can check your blood pressure by means of a simple test using an inflatable arm cuff. Blood pressure often can be entirely controlled by getting regular physical activity, losing excess weight, cutting down on alcohol, and changing eating habits, such as using less salt and other forms of sodium. For some people, medication is also needed.

High Blood Cholesterol. High blood cholesterol can lead to the build-up of plaque in your arteries, which raises the risk of a heart attack. Starting at age 20, everyone should have their cholesterol levels checked by means of a blood test called a "lipoprotein profile." You can lower high blood cholesterol by getting regular physical activity, eating less saturated fat and trans fat, and managing your weight. In some cases, medication is also needed.

Overweight. If you are overweight or obese, you are more likely to develop heart disease even if you have no other risk factors. Ask your doctor to help you determine whether you need to lose weight for your health. The good news? Losing just 5–10 percent of your current weight will help to lower your risk of heart disease and prevent many other medical disorders.

Diabetes greatly increases your risk for heart disease, stroke, and other serious diseases. Ask your doctor whether you should be tested for it. Many people at high risk for diabetes can prevent or delay the disease by reducing calories as part of a healthy eating plan, and by becoming more physically active. If you already have diabetes, work closely with your doctor to manage it.

Moving Toward Health

Becoming physically active may start as a reminder note on your calendar and then become—when you least expect it—a habit and a pleasure. As you strengthen your heart, you may find that getting fit also gives you more energy, stamina, and ability to cope with the ups and downs of daily life. The fact is, getting regular physical activity is one of the single best choices you can make for yourself and your health.

So make the choice today. Go for a walk, a swim, or a bike ride around your neighborhood. Dance, rake leaves, or play tag with a child. Do what you enjoy, and do it regularly. You are helping your health—and burning calories—whenever you are on the move.

Eight Tips for Heart Health

1. Become—and stay—physically active.
2. Balance your calorie intake with the calories you burn in physical activity.
3. Lose weight if you're overweight.
4. If you smoke, stop. Avoid other people's smoke if you can.
5. Control high blood pressure.
6. Control high blood cholesterol.
7. Control diabetes.
8. Choose foods low in saturated fat, *trans* fat, cholesterol, sugar, and salt, especially fruits, vegetables, and whole grains.

The Benefits Keep Coming

It is hard to imagine a single practice with more health benefits than regular physical activity.

In addition to protecting your heart in numerous ways, staying active:

- May help to prevent cancers of the breast, uterus, and colon.
- Strengthens your lungs and helps them to work more efficiently.
- Tones and strengthens your muscles.
- Builds stamina.
- Keeps your joints in good condition.
- Improves balance.
- May slow bone loss.

Regular physical activity can also boost the way you feel. It may:

- Give you more energy.
- Help you to relax and cope better with stress.
- Build confidence.
- Allow you to fall asleep more quickly and sleep more soundly.
- Help you to beat the blues.
- Provide an enjoyable way to share time with friends or family.

Small daily changes will lead to big results over time. A reduction of only 500 calories a day adds up to a weight loss of 25 lbs in six months.

Make a Dash for DASH and Lower Your Blood Pressure

DASH is a diet with proven success in weight loss. But don't forget that it also helps prevent hypertension and will help you fight heart disease and many other health problems. Exercise is so important for overall health and for reducing blood pressure. It is particularly effective when used together with DASH to achieve your ideal calorie balance and reach and maintain your healthy weight.

12

Ready, Set, Go! The Exercise DASH

Getting started

Your physical activity program can be as simple as a 15-minute walk around the block each morning and evening. Gradually build up your program and set new goals to stay motivated. The important thing is to find something you enjoy, and do it safely. And remember trying too hard at first can lead to injury and cause you to give up. Be sure to talk with your doctor before launching any new physical activity program.

___1. **Set a schedule and do your best to keep it.**.

___2. **Get a friend or family member to join you.** Motivate each other to keep it up.

___3. **Cross-train.** Alternate between different activities so you don't strain one part of your body day after day.

___4. **Set goals.** It helps to make your goals clear from the beginning, but to change them as needed.

___5. **Reward yourself.** At the end of each month that you have stayed on your exercise program, reward yourself with something new—new clothes, a compact disc, a movie, a new book—not food, of course, but something you enjoy that will help keep you committed.

By setting smaller goals within your bigger ones, you're less likely to push yourself too hard. Just as important, you give yourself a chance to succeed—over and over.

Set Small Goals. Be Realistic.
Reward Yourself for Progress.

Physical Activity: The Calorie Connection

One way that regular physical activity protects against heart disease is by burning extra calories, which helps you to lose excess weight or stay at your desirable weight. To understand how physical activity affects calories, it is helpful to remember the concept of "energy balance" from Chapter 9. Energy balance is the amount of calories you take in relative to the amount of calories you burn. Per week, you need to burn off about 3,500 more calories than you take in to lose 1 pound. If you need to lose weight, regular physical activity can help you in one of two ways.

First, you can eat your usual amount of calories, but be more active. For example, a 200-pound person who keeps on eating the same amount of calories, but begins to walk briskly each day for 1½ miles, will lose about 14 pounds in 1 year. Staying active will also help to keep the weight off.

Second, you can eat fewer calories and be more active. This is the best way to lose weight, since you're more likely to be successful by combining a healthful, lower-calorie diet with physical activity. For example, a 200-pound person who consumes 250 fewer calories per day, and begins to walk briskly each day for 1½ miles, will lose about 40 pounds in 1 year.

Most of the energy you burn each day—about three quarters of it—goes to activities that your body automatically engages in for survival, such as breathing, sleeping, and digesting food. The part of your energy output that you control is daily physical activity. Any activity you take part in beyond your body's automatic activities will burn extra calories.

Even seated activities, such as using the computer or watching TV, will burn calories—but only a very small number. That is why it is important to make time each day for moderate-to-vigorous physical activity.

Go for the Burn!

Some physical activities burn more calories than others. Below are the average number of calories a 154-pound person will burn, per hour, for a variety of activities. A lighter person will burn fewer calories; a heavier person will burn more. As you can see, vigorous-intensity activities burn more calories than moderate-intensity activities. It is important to choose activities that you like so you are more likely to want to add exercise into your daily routine.

Activities and Calories

Moderate Physical Activity	**Calories Burned per Hour**
Hiking	370
Light gardening/yard work	330
Dancing	330
Golf (walking and carrying clubs)	330
Bicycling (less than 10 mph)	290
Walking (3.5 mph)	280
Weight lifting (light workout)	220
Stretching	180

Vigorous Physical Activity	Calories Burned per Hour
Running/jogging	590
Bicycling (more than 10 mph)	590
Swimming (slow freestyle laps)	510
Aerobics	480
Walking (4.5 mph)	460
Heavy yard work (chopping wood, for example)	440
Weight lifting (vigorous workout)	440
Basketball (vigorous)	440

Source: Adapted from the 2005 Dietary Guidelines Advisory Committee Report

75% of Your Daily Calories is Used for Survival

Most of the energy you burn each day—about three quarters of it—goes to activities that your body automatically engages in for survival, such as breathing, sleeping, and digesting food.

The part of your energy output that you control is daily physical activity. Any activity you take part in beyond your body's automatic activities will burn extra calories. Even seated activities, such as using the computer or watching TV, will burn calories—but only a very small number.

That's why it's important to make time each day for moderate-to-vigorous physical activity.

Before You Begin

- If your blood pressure is moderately high, 30 minutes of brisk walking on most days a week may be enough to keep you off of medication.
- If you take medication for high blood pressure, 30 minutes of moderate physical activity can make your medication work more effectively and make you feel better.
- If you don't have high blood pressure, being physically active can help keep it that way. If you have normal blood pressure—but are not active—your chances of developing high blood pressure increase, especially as you get older or if you become overweight or obese or develop diabetes.

Great Moves

Given the numerous benefits of regular physical activity, you may be ready to begin. But first, it is good to understand how activities differ from one another and how each form of movement uniquely contributes to your health. Three types of activity are important for a complete physical activity program: aerobic activity, resistance training, and flexibility exercises. Let's take a brief look at each one.

Three types of activity are important for a complete physical activity program: aerobic activity, resistance training, and flexibility exercises.

Types of Physical Activity

Aerobic activity is any physical activity that uses large muscle groups and causes your body to use more oxygen than it would while resting.

Aerobic activity is the type of movement that most benefits the heart. Examples of aerobic activity are brisk walking, jogging, and bicycling.

Resistance training—is also called strength training and it can firm, strengthen, and tone your muscles, as well as improve your bone strength, balance, and coordination. Examples of strength moves are pushups, lunges, and bicep curls using dumbbells.

Flexibility exercises—these stretch and lengthen your muscles. Flexibility activities help to improve joint flexibility and keep muscles limber, thereby preventing injury. An example of a stretching move is sitting cross-legged on the floor and gently pushing down on the tops of your legs to stretch the inner thigh muscles.

Working Together for Health

While aerobic activities benefit the heart most, all three types of movement are vital components of a physical activity program. They also work together in important ways. For example, resistance exercises can help you achieve the muscle strength, balance, and coordination to do your aerobic activities more successfully. Meanwhile, flexibility training will help you to move your muscles and joints more easily and prevent injury as you engage in aerobic activities.

Keep in mind, too, that you can break up any activity into shorter periods of at least 10 minutes each. For example, if you want to total 30 minutes of activity per day, you could spend 10 minutes walking on your lunch break, another 10 minutes raking leaves in the backyard, and another 10 minutes lifting weights.

Small daily changes will lead to big results over time. A reduction of only 500 calories a day adds up to a weight loss of 25 lbs in six months.

Remember the Benefits: In Chapter 11 you read how regular physical activity has many benefits. It can:

- Give you more energy.
- Help you to relax and cope better with stress.
- Build confidence.
- Allow you to fall asleep more quickly and sleep more soundly.
- Help you to beat the blues.
- Provide an enjoyable way to share time with friends or family.

A Complete Activity Program

A Sample Weekly Schedule

Sunday	Aerobic		Stretch
Monday	Aerobic	Strength	Stretch
Tuesday	Aerobic		Stretch
Wednesday	Aerobic	Strength	Stretch
Thursday	Aerobic		Stretch
Friday	Aerobic	Strength	Stretch
Saturday	Aerobic		Stretch

Three Moves for Health

While not usually aerobic, the activities below offer numerous health benefits and are enjoyable ways to get and stay in shape. All are offered at many YMCAs, community centers, and gyms.

Yoga is a system of physical postures, stretching, and breathing techniques that can improve flexibility, balance, muscle strength, and relaxation. Many styles are available, ranging from slow and gentle to athletic and vigorous. A recent study found that regular yoga practice may help to minimize weight gain in middle age.

Tai chi is an ancient Chinese practice that shifts your body weight as you go through a series of slow movements that flow rhythmically together into one graceful gesture. This gentle, calming practice can help to improve flexibility, balance and muscle strength.

Pilates is a body conditioning routine that seeks to strengthen the body's "core" (torso), usually through a series of mat exercises. Another Pilates method uses special exercise machines, available at some health clubs. It can strengthen and tone muscles as well as increase flexibility.

Intensity Levels

Generally, the more vigorously you engage in an activity, and the more time you spend doing it, the more health benefits you will receive. The vigorous activities listed in the left column of the box, "Choosing Your Moves," are especially helpful for conditioning your heart and lungs, and these activities also burn more calories than those that are less vigorous.

However, moderate-intensity activities can also be excellent fitness choices. When done briskly for 30 minutes or longer on most days of the week, the moderate-intensity activities listed in the column on the right side of the box can help to condition your heart and lungs and reduce your risk of heart disease.

Choosing Your Moves

Vigorous activity	**Moderate activity**
Aerobic dancing	Bicycling (less than 10 mph)
Basketball	Downhill skiing
Bicycling (more than 10 mph)	Dancing
Cross-country skiing	Gardening
Hiking (uphill)	Golf (on foot)
Ice hockey/field hockey	Hiking (flat ground)
Jogging/running (at least 5 mph)	Horseback riding
Jumping rope	Roller skating/ice skating
Soccer	Softball
Stair climbing	Swimming
Tennis (singles)	Tennis (doubles)
Walking briskly (4.5 mph)	Walking moderately (3.5 mph)
Yard work (heavy)	Yard work (light)

Taking Precautions

It is wise to get medical advice before starting, or significantly increasing, physical activity. Check with your doctor first if you:

- Are over 50 years old and not used to moderately energetic activity.
- Currently have a heart condition, have developed chest pain within the last month, or have had a heart attack. (Also see the section, "After a Heart Attack.")
- Have a parent or sibling who developed heart disease at an early age.
- Have any other chronic health problem or risk factors for a chronic disease.
- Tend to easily lose your balance or become dizzy.
- Feel extremely breathless after mild exertion.
- Are on any type of medication.

Check with your doctor before increasing physical activity or beginning a diet.

How Do I Know If I'm Exercising Too Much or Too Little?

Unless you're in excellent physical condition, any physical activity that boosts your heart rate above 75 percent of your maximum rate is likely to be too strenuous.

By the same token, any activity that increases your heart rate to less than 50 percent of your maximum rate gives your heart and lungs too little conditioning.

The most healthful activity level uses 50–75 percent of your maximum heart rate. This range, called your target heart rate zone, is shown in the table on page 125. During the first few months of your activity program, aim to reach 50 percent of your maximum rate. As you get into better shape, you can slowly build up to 75 percent.

Keep in mind that "getting into the zone" doesn't mean pushing yourself to the limit. For example, while walking briskly or jogging, you should be able to keep up a conversation without trouble. If you can't, move a bit more slowly. Overall, a gentle, gradual approach will help you to maximize your gains and minimize your risks.

Take Your Pulse – Wrist or Neck

To find out whether you're within your target heart rate zone, take your pulse immediately after finishing your activity. Here's how:

- As soon as you stop your activity, place the tips of your first two fingers lightly over one of the two blood vessels on your neck, located to the left and right of your Adam's apple.

- Another convenient pulse spot is on the inside of your wrist, just below the base of your thumb. Put your fingers (not your thumb on your wrist) so that you can feel your pulse beating. Count your pulse for 10 seconds and multiply by six. (e.g. 12 x 6 = a resting pulse of 72)

- Count your pulse for 10 seconds and multiply by six. (e.g. 12 x 6 = 72)

- If your pulse falls within your target zone, your activity is providing good benefits for your heart and lungs. If you're below your target heart rate zone, move just a bit faster next time, as long as you continue to feel reasonably comfortable doing so. If you're above your target zone, move a little more slowly. Don't try to move at, or very close to, your maximum heart rate—that's working too hard.

- Eventually, you'll be consistently engaging in your activity within your target zone. To continue to track your progress, keep checking your pulse after at least one activity session per week.

Measuring Your Heart Rate:

Count your pulse for 10 seconds and multiply by six.
Pulse for 10 seconds x 6 = ______
This gives you your heart rate in a minute.

Date: ____________________

My Resting Pulse:_________

Tracking Your Target Heart Rate

As you become more physically active, how will you know whether you're improving your heart and lung fitness? The best way is to track your target heart rate during your activity. Your target heart rate is a percentage of your maximum heart rate, which is the fastest your heart can beat, based on your age. See the chart on page 125 to find your own target heart rate.

What's Your Target Heart Rate?

To find your target heart rate zone, look for the age closest to yours in the table on the next page. For example, if you're 40, your target zone is 90–135 beats per minute. If you're 53, the closest age on the chart is 55, so your target zone is 83–123 beats per minute. Be aware that the figures in the table are averages, so use them as general guidelines.

Find Your Target Heart Rate Zone

Age	**Target Heart Rate Zone: 50–75%**	**Maximum Heart Rate: 100%**
20	100–150 beats per min.	200 beats per min.
25	98–146 beats per min.	195 beats per min.
30	95–142 beats per min.	190 beats per min.
35	93–138 beats per min.	185 beats per min.
40	90–135 beats per min.	180 beats per min.
45	88–131 beats per min.	175 beats per min.
50	85–127 beats per min.	170 beats per min.
55	83–123 beats per min.	165 beats per min.
60	80–120 beats per min.	160 beats per min.
65	78–116 beats per min.	155 beats per min.
70	75–113 beats per min.	150 beats per min.

Date: __________

My resting pulse __________

My target heart rate __________

Gradually build up your program and set new goals to stay motivated. The important thing is to find something you enjoy, and do it safely.

Remember (and this is contingent on your doctor's advice):

Too much. Unless you're in excellent physical condition, any physical activity that boosts your heart rate above 75 percent of your maximum rate is likely to be too strenuous.

Too little. By the same token, any activity that increases your heart rate to less than 50 percent of your maximum rate gives your heart and lungs too little conditioning. The first few months: aim to reach 50 percent of your maximum rate.

As you build stamina gradually increase your exercise to boost your heart rate up to 75 percent.

> **The first few months: aim to reach 50 percent of your maximum rate. As you build stamina, gradually increase up to 75 percent.**

Getting in Motion

Ready to get moving? If so, getting health benefits from regular activity may be easier than you think. As discussed at the start of this book, about 30 minutes of moderate-intensity physical activity on most—and preferably all—days of the week will help you to reduce the risk of heart disease. If you can gradually work up to more time being active, you'll get even more benefits.

Brisk walking is a simple, enjoyable way to help keep your heart healthy. One study showed that regular, brisk walking reduced the risk of heart attack by the same amount as more vigorous exercise, such as jogging. And it is possible to walk when the weather is bad; many people now go to a nearby mall to exercise indoors.

Most physical activities don't require any special athletic skills. In addition to walking, some examples of activities that many people do regularly are biking, gardening, tennis, dancing, or swimming. Some people prefer to use simple exercise equipment at home or they find the gym environment to be a more motivating place. The important thing is to find the activities you like to do—and to stay active.

All adults should add at least 30 minutes of moderate-intensity physical activity to their daily routine on most days of the week. To prevent weight gain, some people may need 60 minutes of moderate- to vigorous-intensity activity on most days of the week, while not eating more calories than needed for their basic activity level.

Even 20 minutes a day of walking, divided into two 10 minute segments, can yield health benefits. If you are unable to exercise for 30 minutes every day, then try to walk for 20-30 minutes, even if it is broken up into two sessions. The most important thing is to not be sedentary. Remember, to lose weight you need to cut calories below your daily needs or increase energy burned beyond your basic daily needs. If you do both, you will lose weight faster while at the same time building your muscle tone which also will help with weight loss.

Brisk walking is a convenient and heart-healthy activity.

Questionnaire: Choosing the Right Activity

The key to a successful fitness program is choosing an activity or activities that will work well for you. Here are some questions to ask yourself to help you find a good "movement match."

1. How physically fit are you?

1. **___ I exercise regularly and am very fit.**
2. **___ I exercise a couple of times a week. Good in some ways.**
3. **___ I'm busy, but don't get much structured exercise. Not very fit.**
4. **___ I exercise infrequently or not at all. Very out-of-shape.**

If you haven't exercised for a while, the good news is that it's not too late to start. And, if you're out of shape, you will begin to see improvement in the way you look and feel even faster than someone who habitually exercises. .

2. Do you prefer to be active on your own, or with others?

____ on my own
____ with others

Do you like individual activities, such as swimming or weight lifting; two-person activities, such as dancing? Or do you prefer group sports, such as softball or doubles tennis? If you like to be active with others, consider whether you can find a partner or group easily and quickly. If not, choose another activity until you can find a partner.

Choosing an activity you truly enjoy and can easily schedule will help you to commit to an activity program and to stay with it.

3. Would you rather do activities outdoors or in your home?

___outdoors ___at home

4. How does cost affect your choice of activity? I prefer. . .

___Free activities. For example, brisk walking requires only a comfortable pair of rubber-soled shoes. Many communities also offer free or very affordable physical activity options. Check with your local park and recreation department, which may offer a number of low-cost physical activity classes that are enjoyable for the entire family. There are also current game platforms—Nintendo, X-Box, Playstation, and others—that have games, sports and dancing activities that can improve your fitness in an enjoyable way. Of course, they require a small initial purchase, but then can be done in the comfort of your home any time you like. Many inexpensive dvds also have a variety of exercise activities.

___**Gym, club or trainer.** Some people find that regularly going to a health club, and/or working with a fitness trainer, helps them to stay more motivated. Before you purchase a gym membership or sessions with a professional, be sure to shop around and ask questions.

Do more of the activities you already like and already know how to do.

5. Based on my answers above and other information in this chapter, I think these would be good choices for my daily exercise: ____

____

6. I plan to exercise __every day or __3-4 times a week.

How long: ____

When: ____

Where: ____

One mile equals roughly 2,000 steps, or 15 minutes of physical activity.

2000 steps = 1 mile = 15 minutes at a good pace

Creating Opportunities

It's easier to stay physically active over time if you take advantage of everyday opportunities to move around. For example:

- Use the stairs—both up and down—instead of the elevator. Start with one flight of stairs and gradually build up to more.
- Walk more. Park a few blocks from the office or store and walk the rest of the way. If you take public transportation, get off a stop or two early and walk a few blocks.
- While working, take frequent activity breaks. Get up and stretch, walk around, and give your muscles and mind a chance to relax.
- Instead of eating that extra snack, take a brisk stroll around the neighborhood or your office building.
- Do housework, gardening, or yard work at a more vigorous pace.
- When you travel, walk around the train station, bus station, or airport rather than sitting and waiting.
- Keep moving while you watch TV. Lift hand weights, do some gentle yoga stretches, or pedal an exercise bike.
- Better yet, turn off the TV and take a brisk walk.

It's Time to Begin...

In the past chapters, you've made an individual profile of your weight, health and fitness. You've read about the benefits of DASH and physical activity, and made a commitment to lose weight and get healthier with regular exercise. You've analyzed your activity level and daily calorie needs. You've looked at the DASH daily servings and how they represent different daily calorie counts.

The next chapter gives you the opportunity to look over all that you have learned about yourself and DASH. This will help as you begin your *60 day Weight Loss and Fitness Journal.*

13

Review: You and DASH

Today's Date: ________________

My weight __________

My BMI (p.20) __________

My blood pressure (p.33) __________

It is (circle one): Normal Prehypertension High

My Cholesterol (p.51) __________

LDL __________

HDL __________

Triglycerides __________

My resting pulse (p.123) __________

My target heart rate (p.125) __________

My lifestyle (p.70) sedentary moderately active active

My calorie needs (p.71) __________

Sodium goal per day: __________ mg.

How will I add potassium to my diet? (pp.45-48)

____

Two eating habits I will change:

____

____

My choice(s) of exercise (p.128-129):

____

____

# of minutes I plan to exercise a day: ________________

When I will exercise (times/days):

____

Optional Measurements

While you are dieting and exercising, your body will be losing weight and gaining muscle. At times you may see results faster in your changing measurements (and in the way your clothing fits) than you do by looking at your weight on a scale. This page will be useful if you would like to keep a records with a tape measure and compare them at different dates.

Date: **Date:** **Date:**

____

Waist ______________________________

Bust ______________________________

Hips ______________________________

Upper arm ______________________________

Upper thigh ______________________________

Clothing size

Men: shirt: ______________________________

trousers: ______________________________

jeans ______________________________

jacket ______________________________

suit: ______________________________

Women: size: ______________________________

slacks ______________________________

jeans ______________________________

blouse/shirt: ______________________________

dress: ______________________________

other (swimsuit, etc): ______________________________

14

The DASH Journal

Your 60-Day Diet Journal

14

60 Day DASH Journal

Track your progress here every week:

Date: __________

My weight __________
My blood pressure __________

Date: __________

My weight __________
My blood pressure __________

Date: __________

My weight __________
My blood pressure __________

Date: __________

My weight __________
My blood pressure __________

Date: __________

My weight __________
My blood pressure __________

Date: __________

My weight __________
My blood pressure __________

*If you do not have a blood pressure cuff, most drugstores and pharmacies have them available to the public for free.

Date: ___________

My weight ___________
My blood pressure ___________

Date: ___________

My weight ___________
My blood pressure ___________

Date: ___________

My weight ___________
My blood pressure ___________

Date: ___________

My weight ___________
My blood pressure ___________

Date: ___________

My weight ___________
My blood pressure ___________

Date: ___________

My weight ___________
My blood pressure ___________

Date: ___________

My weight ___________
My blood pressure ___________

Date: ___________

My weight ___________
My blood pressure ___________

Remember the DASH Basics

How to Lose Weight, Lower Blood Pressure and Get Healthy with DASH

1. Keep a Healthy Blood Pressure
2. Reduce Sodium/Salt to ¾ tsp – 1 tsp a day.
3. Eat Potassium-rich Foods
4. Lean Meat – Fruits – Vegetables – Whole Grains – Milk
5. Cut Back on Processed Foods
6. Keep a Healthy BMI
7. Exercise 30 minutes a day
8. Keep a Diet Journal

To make it easiy to count your daily servings, here again are the four most common calorie plans (easily adjusted with servings of protein, dairy and/or grain). Every day's Dash journal page also includes a copy of the plan for 2000 calories, for your convenient reference.

The Daily DASH Diet
1600 calories

Food Groups	Servings
Grains*	6
Vegetables	3 - 4
Fruits	4
Milk and milk products, fat-free or lowfat	**2 - 3**
Lean meats, poultry, and fish	3 - 6
Nuts, seeds, and legumes	3/week
Fats and oils	2
Sweets and added sugars	0

*Whole grains are recommended for most grain servings as a good source of fiber and nutrients.

The Daily DASH Diet
2000 calories

Food Groups	Servings
Grains*	6 - 8
Vegetables	4 - 5
Fruits	4 - 5
Milk and milk products, fat-free or lowfat	2 - 3
Lean meats, poultry, and fish	6 or less
Nuts, seeds, and legumes	4 - 5/week
Fats and oils	2 - 3
Sweets and added sugars	≤2

*Whole grains are recommended for most grain servings as a good source of fiber and nutrients.

The Daily DASH Diet
2600 calories

Food Groups	Servings
Grains*	10 - 11
Vegetables	5 - 6
Fruits	5 - 6
Milk and milk products, fat-free or lowfat	3
Lean meats, poultry, and fish	6
Nuts, seeds, and legumes	1
Fats and oils	2 - 3
Sweets and added sugars	3

*Whole grains are recommended for most grain servings as a good source of fiber and nutrients.

The Daily DASH Diet
3100 calories

Food Groups	Servings
Grains*	12 - 13
Vegetables	6
Fruits	6
Milk and milk products, fat-free or lowfat	3 - 4
Lean meats, poultry, and fish	6 - 9
Nuts, seeds, and legumes	1
Fats and oils	2 - 3
Sweets and added sugars	4

*Whole grains are recommended for most grain servings as a good source of fiber and nutrients.

Here is a review of the DASH serving sizes.

Food Groups	Serving Size
Grains*	bread 1 slice cereal†, 1 oz dry rice, pasta, or cereal, ½ cup
Vegetables	raw leafy, 1 cup cut-up raw or cooked, ½ cup vegetable juice, ½ cup
Fruits	1 medium dried fruit, ¼ cup fresh, frozen, or canned, ½ cup fruit juice, ½ cup
Milk products (low fat or non fat)	milk or yogurt, 1 cup cheese, 1 ½ oz.
Meats, fish and poultry	cooked, 1 oz 1 egg‡
Nuts, seeds, and legumes	nuts, ⅓ cup or 1 ½ oz. 2 Tbsp peanut butter 2 Tbsp or ½ oz. seeds ½ cup cooked legumes (dry beans and peas)
Fats and oil	1 tsp soft margarine

DAY 1 Date: ___________

Time	Food	Comments

6-8 8 oz. glasses of water √ ☐ ☐ ☐ ☐ ☐ ☐ ☐ ☐

Exercise? ☐ **Yes** ☐ **No** _________ **minutes**

Exercise/Activity:

____

____

The Daily DASH Diet
2000 Calorie Plan (reduce or add food as needed)
Sodium Goal: 2300 mg/day or 1500 mg/day

Grains – 4-6 servings per day; try for whole grains
☐ ☐ ☐ ☐ ☐ ☐

Vegetables – 4-6 servings per day; (serving = ½ c)
☐ ☐ ☐ ☐ ☐ ☐

Fruit – 4-6 servings per day; (serving= ½ c.)
☐ ☐ ☐ ☐ ☐ ☐

Milk & Milk Products – 2-3 servings (serving = 8 oz)
☐ ☐ ☐

Meat, Chicken, Fish – 6 servings (1 serving =1oz)
☐ ☐ ☐ ☐ ☐ ☐

Nuts, seeds, and legumes -- 4–5 per week
☐ ☐ ☐ ☐ ☐ ☐

Fats and oils – 2-3 per day
☐ ☐ ☐

Sweets and sugar – 5 servings or less per week
☐ ☐ ☐ ☐ ☐

How did you do today? √

A great day ☐ **Mostly followed DASH**☐ **I'll do better tomorrow** ☐

Your thoughts and feelings about dieting so far:

____

____

____

DAY **2** Date: ___________

Time	Food	Comments

6-8 8 oz. glasses of water √ ☐ ☐ ☐ ☐ ☐ ☐ ☐ ☐

Exercise? ☐ **Yes** ☐ **No** _________ **minutes**

Exercise/Activity:

____

____

The Daily DASH Diet
2000 Calorie Plan (reduce or add food as needed)
Sodium Goal: 2300 mg/day or 1500 mg/day

Grains – 4-6 servings per day; try for whole grains
☐ ☐ ☐ ☐ ☐ ☐

Vegetables – 4-6 servings per day; (serving = ½ c)
☐ ☐ ☐ ☐ ☐ ☐

Fruit – 4-6 servings per day; (serving= ½ c.)
☐ ☐ ☐ ☐ ☐ ☐

Milk & Milk Products – 2-3 servings (serving = 8 oz)
☐ ☐ ☐

Meat, Chicken, Fish – 6 servings (1 serving =1oz)
☐ ☐ ☐ ☐ ☐ ☐

Nuts, seeds, and legumes -- 4–5 per week
☐ ☐ ☐ ☐ ☐ ☐

Fats and oils – 2-3 per day
☐ ☐ ☐

Sweets and sugar – 5 servings or less per week
☐ ☐ ☐ ☐ ☐

How did you do today? √

A great day ☐ **Mostly followed DASH**☐ **I'll do better tomorrow** ☐

Your thoughts and feelings about dieting so far:

____

____

____

DAY **3** Date: ___________

Time	Food	Comments

6-8 8 oz. glasses of water √ ☐ ☐ ☐ ☐ ☐ ☐ ☐ ☐

Exercise? ☐ **Yes** ☐ **No** _________ **minutes**

Exercise/Activity:

____

____

The Daily DASH Diet
2000 Calorie Plan (reduce or add food as needed)
Sodium Goal: 2300 mg/day or 1500 mg/day

Grains – 4-6 servings per day; try for whole grains
☐ ☐ ☐ ☐ ☐ ☐

Vegetables – 4-6 servings per day; (serving = ½ c)
☐ ☐ ☐ ☐ ☐ ☐

Fruit – 4-6 servings per day; (serving= ½ c.)
☐ ☐ ☐ ☐ ☐ ☐

Milk & Milk Products – 2-3 servings (serving = 8 oz)
☐ ☐ ☐

Meat, Chicken, Fish – 6 servings (1 serving =1oz)
☐ ☐ ☐ ☐ ☐ ☐

Nuts, seeds, and legumes -- 4–5 per week
☐ ☐ ☐ ☐ ☐ ☐

Fats and oils – 2-3 per day
☐ ☐ ☐

Sweets and sugar – 5 servings or less per week
☐ ☐ ☐ ☐ ☐

How did you do today? √

A great day ☐ **Mostly followed DASH**☐ **I'll do better tomorrow** ☐

Your thoughts and feelings about dieting so far:

____

____

____

DAY 4 **Date: ___________**

Time	Food	Comments

6-8 8 oz. glasses of water √ ☐ ☐ ☐ ☐ ☐ ☐ ☐ ☐

Exercise? ☐ **Yes** ☐ **No** _________ **minutes**

Exercise/Activity:

____

____

The Daily DASH Diet
2000 Calorie Plan (reduce or add food as needed)
Sodium Goal: 2300 mg/day or 1500 mg/day

Grains – 4-6 servings per day; try for whole grains
☐ ☐ ☐ ☐ ☐ ☐

Vegetables – 4-6 servings per day; (serving = ½ c)
☐ ☐ ☐ ☐ ☐ ☐

Fruit – 4-6 servings per day; (serving= ½ c.)
☐ ☐ ☐ ☐ ☐ ☐

Milk & Milk Products – 2-3 servings (serving = 8 oz)
☐ ☐ ☐

Meat, Chicken, Fish – 6 servings (1 serving =1oz)
☐ ☐ ☐ ☐ ☐ ☐

Nuts, seeds, and legumes -- 4–5 per week
☐ ☐ ☐ ☐ ☐ ☐

Fats and oils – 2-3 per day
☐ ☐ ☐

Sweets and sugar – 5 servings or less per week
☐ ☐ ☐ ☐ ☐

How did you do today? √

A great day ☐ **Mostly followed DASH**☐ **I'll do better tomorrow** ☐

Your thoughts and feelings about dieting so far:

____

____

____

DAY 5 Date: ____________

Time	Food	Comments

6-8 8 oz. glasses of water √ ☐ ☐ ☐ ☐ ☐ ☐ ☐ ☐

Exercise? ☐ **Yes** ☐ **No** _________ **minutes**

Exercise/Activity:

____

____

The Daily DASH Diet
2000 Calorie Plan (reduce or add food as needed)
Sodium Goal: 2300 mg/day or 1500 mg/day

Grains – 4-6 servings per day; try for whole grains
☐ ☐ ☐ ☐ ☐ ☐

Vegetables – 4-6 servings per day; (serving = ½ c)
☐ ☐ ☐ ☐ ☐ ☐

Fruit – 4-6 servings per day; (serving= ½ c.)
☐ ☐ ☐ ☐ ☐ ☐

Milk & Milk Products – 2-3 servings (serving = 8 oz)
☐ ☐ ☐

Meat, Chicken, Fish – 6 servings (1 serving =1oz)
☐ ☐ ☐ ☐ ☐ ☐

Nuts, seeds, and legumes -- 4–5 per week
☐ ☐ ☐ ☐ ☐ ☐

Fats and oils – 2-3 per day
☐ ☐ ☐

Sweets and sugar – 5 servings or less per week
☐ ☐ ☐ ☐ ☐

How did you do today? √

A great day ☐ **Mostly followed DASH**☐ **I'll do better tomorrow** ☐

Your thoughts and feelings about dieting so far:

____

____

____

DAY 6 Date: ____________

Time	Food	Comments

6-8 8 oz. glasses of water √ ☐ ☐ ☐ ☐ ☐ ☐ ☐ ☐

Exercise? ☐ **Yes** ☐ **No** _________ **minutes**

Exercise/Activity:

____

____

The Daily DASH Diet
2000 Calorie Plan (reduce or add food as needed)
Sodium Goal: 2300 mg/day or 1500 mg/day

Grains – 4-6 servings per day; try for whole grains
☐ ☐ ☐ ☐ ☐ ☐

Vegetables – 4-6 servings per day; (serving = ½ c)
☐ ☐ ☐ ☐ ☐ ☐

Fruit – 4-6 servings per day; (serving= ½ c.)
☐ ☐ ☐ ☐ ☐ ☐

Milk & Milk Products – 2-3 servings (serving = 8 oz)
☐ ☐ ☐

Meat, Chicken, Fish – 6 servings (1 serving =1oz)
☐ ☐ ☐ ☐ ☐ ☐

Nuts, seeds, and legumes -- 4–5 per week
☐ ☐ ☐ ☐ ☐ ☐

Fats and oils – 2-3 per day
☐ ☐ ☐

Sweets and sugar – 5 servings or less per week
☐ ☐ ☐ ☐ ☐

How did you do today? √

A great day ☐ **Mostly followed DASH**☐ **I'll do better tomorrow** ☐

Your thoughts and feelings about dieting so far:

____

____

____

DAY 7 **Date: ___________**

Time	Food	Comments

6-8 8 oz. glasses of water √ ☐ ☐ ☐ ☐ ☐ ☐ ☐ ☐

Exercise? ☐ **Yes** ☐ **No** _________ **minutes**

Exercise/Activity:

____

____

The Daily DASH Diet
2000 Calorie Plan (reduce or add food as needed)
Sodium Goal: 2300 mg/day or 1500 mg/day

Grains – 4-6 servings per day; try for whole grains
☐ ☐ ☐ ☐ ☐ ☐

Vegetables – 4-6 servings per day; (serving = ½ c)
☐ ☐ ☐ ☐ ☐ ☐

Fruit – 4-6 servings per day; (serving= ½ c.)
☐ ☐ ☐ ☐ ☐ ☐

Milk & Milk Products – 2-3 servings (serving = 8 oz)
☐ ☐ ☐

Meat, Chicken, Fish – 6 servings (1 serving =1oz)
☐ ☐ ☐ ☐ ☐ ☐

Nuts, seeds, and legumes -- 4–5 per week
☐ ☐ ☐ ☐ ☐ ☐

Fats and oils – 2-3 per day
☐ ☐ ☐

Sweets and sugar – 5 servings or less per week
☐ ☐ ☐ ☐ ☐

How did you do today? √

A great day ☐ **Mostly followed DASH**☐ **I'll do better tomorrow** ☐

Your thoughts and feelings about dieting so far:

____

____

____

DAY **8** **Date:** ____________

Time	Food	Comments

6-8 8 oz. glasses of water √ ☐ ☐ ☐ ☐ ☐ ☐ ☐ ☐

Exercise? ☐ **Yes** ☐ **No** _________ **minutes**

Exercise/Activity:

____

____

The Daily DASH Diet
2000 Calorie Plan (reduce or add food as needed)
Sodium Goal: 2300 mg/day or 1500 mg/day

Grains – 4-6 servings per day; try for whole grains
☐ ☐ ☐ ☐ ☐ ☐
Vegetables – 4-6 servings per day; (serving = ½ c)
☐ ☐ ☐ ☐ ☐ ☐
Fruit – 4-6 servings per day; (serving= ½ c.)
☐ ☐ ☐ ☐ ☐ ☐
Milk & Milk Products – 2-3 servings (serving = 8 oz)
☐ ☐ ☐
Meat, Chicken, Fish – 6 servings (1 serving =1oz)
☐ ☐ ☐ ☐ ☐ ☐
Nuts, seeds, and legumes -- 4–5 per week
☐ ☐ ☐ ☐ ☐ ☐
Fats and oils – 2-3 per day
☐ ☐ ☐
Sweets and sugar – 5 servings or less per week
☐ ☐ ☐ ☐ ☐

How did you do today? √

A great day ☐ **Mostly followed DASH**☐ **I'll do better tomorrow** ☐

Your thoughts and feelings about dieting so far:

____

____

____

DAY 9 **Date: ____________**

Time	Food	Comments

6-8 8 oz. glasses of water √ ☐ ☐ ☐ ☐ ☐ ☐ ☐ ☐

Exercise? ☐ **Yes** ☐ **No** _________ **minutes**

Exercise/Activity:

____

____

The Daily DASH Diet
2000 Calorie Plan (reduce or add food as needed)
Sodium Goal: 2300 mg/day or 1500 mg/day

Grains – 4-6 servings per day; try for whole grains
☐ ☐ ☐ ☐ ☐ ☐

Vegetables – 4-6 servings per day; (serving = ½ c)
☐ ☐ ☐ ☐ ☐ ☐

Fruit – 4-6 servings per day; (serving= ½ c.)
☐ ☐ ☐ ☐ ☐ ☐

Milk & Milk Products – 2-3 servings (serving = 8 oz)
☐ ☐ ☐

Meat, Chicken, Fish – 6 servings (1 serving =1oz)
☐ ☐ ☐ ☐ ☐ ☐

Nuts, seeds, and legumes -- 4–5 per week
☐ ☐ ☐ ☐ ☐ ☐

Fats and oils – 2-3 per day
☐ ☐ ☐

Sweets and sugar – 5 servings or less per week
☐ ☐ ☐ ☐ ☐

How did you do today? √

A great day ☐ **Mostly followed DASH**☐ **I'll do better tomorrow** ☐

Your thoughts and feelings about dieting so far:

____

____

____

DAY 10

Date: ____________

Time	Food	Comments

6-8 8 oz. glasses of water √ ☐ ☐ ☐ ☐ ☐ ☐ ☐ ☐

Exercise? ☐ **Yes** ☐ **No** _________ **minutes**

Exercise/Activity:

____

____

The Daily DASH Diet
2000 Calorie Plan (reduce or add food as needed)
Sodium Goal: 2300 mg/day or 1500 mg/day

Grains – 4-6 servings per day; try for whole grains
☐ ☐ ☐ ☐ ☐ ☐
Vegetables – 4-6 servings per day; (serving = ½ c)
☐ ☐ ☐ ☐ ☐ ☐
Fruit – 4-6 servings per day; (serving= ½ c.)
☐ ☐ ☐ ☐ ☐ ☐
Milk & Milk Products – 2-3 servings (serving = 8 oz)
☐ ☐ ☐
Meat, Chicken, Fish – 6 servings (1 serving =1oz)
☐ ☐ ☐ ☐ ☐ ☐
Nuts, seeds, and legumes -- 4–5 per week
☐ ☐ ☐ ☐ ☐ ☐
Fats and oils – 2-3 per day
☐ ☐ ☐
Sweets and sugar – 5 servings or less per week
☐ ☐ ☐ ☐ ☐

How did you do today? √

A great day ☐ **Mostly followed DASH**☐ **I'll do better tomorrow** ☐

Your thoughts and feelings about dieting so far:

____

____

____

DAY 11

Date: ___________

Time	Food	Comments

6-8 8 oz. glasses of water √ ☐ ☐ ☐ ☐ ☐ ☐ ☐ ☐

Exercise? ☐ **Yes** ☐ **No** _________ **minutes**

Exercise/Activity:

____

____

The Daily DASH Diet
2000 Calorie Plan (reduce or add food as needed)
Sodium Goal: 2300 mg/day or 1500 mg/day

Grains – 4-6 servings per day; try for whole grains
☐ ☐ ☐ ☐ ☐ ☐

Vegetables – 4-6 servings per day; (serving = ½ c)
☐ ☐ ☐ ☐ ☐ ☐

Fruit – 4-6 servings per day; (serving= ½ c.)
☐ ☐ ☐ ☐ ☐ ☐

Milk & Milk Products – 2-3 servings (serving = 8 oz)
☐ ☐ ☐

Meat, Chicken, Fish – 6 servings (1 serving =1oz)
☐ ☐ ☐ ☐ ☐ ☐

Nuts, seeds, and legumes -- 4–5 per week
☐ ☐ ☐ ☐ ☐ ☐

Fats and oils – 2-3 per day
☐ ☐ ☐

Sweets and sugar – 5 servings or less per week
☐ ☐ ☐ ☐ ☐

How did you do today? √

A great day ☐ **Mostly followed DASH**☐ **I'll do better tomorrow** ☐

Your thoughts and feelings about dieting so far:

____

____

____

DAY 12 Date: ___________

Time	Food	Comments

6-8 8 oz. glasses of water √ ☐ ☐ ☐ ☐ ☐ ☐ ☐ ☐

Exercise? ☐ **Yes** ☐ **No** ________ **minutes**

Exercise/Activity:

____

____

The Daily DASH Diet

2000 Calorie Plan (reduce or add food as needed)

Sodium Goal: 2300 mg/day or 1500 mg/day

Grains – 4-6 servings per day; try for whole grains

☐ ☐ ☐ ☐ ☐ ☐

Vegetables – 4-6 servings per day; (serving = ½ c)

☐ ☐ ☐ ☐ ☐ ☐

Fruit – 4-6 servings per day; (serving= ½ c.)

☐ ☐ ☐ ☐ ☐ ☐

Milk & Milk Products – 2-3 servings (serving = 8 oz)

☐ ☐ ☐

Meat, Chicken, Fish – 6 servings (1 serving =1oz)

☐ ☐ ☐ ☐ ☐ ☐

Nuts, seeds, and legumes -- 4–5 per week

☐ ☐ ☐ ☐ ☐ ☐

Fats and oils – 2-3 per day

☐ ☐ ☐

Sweets and sugar – 5 servings or less per week

☐ ☐ ☐ ☐ ☐

How did you do today? √

A great day ☐ **Mostly followed DASH**☐ **I'll do better tomorrow** ☐

Your thoughts and feelings about dieting so far:

____

____

____

DAY 13

Date: ____________

Time	Food	Comments

6-8 8 oz. glasses of water √ ☐ ☐ ☐ ☐ ☐ ☐ ☐ ☐

Exercise? ☐ **Yes** ☐ **No** _________ **minutes**

Exercise/Activity:

____

____

The Daily DASH Diet
2000 Calorie Plan (reduce or add food as needed)
Sodium Goal: 2300 mg/day or 1500 mg/day

Grains – 4-6 servings per day; try for whole grains
☐ ☐ ☐ ☐ ☐ ☐

Vegetables – 4-6 servings per day; (serving = ½ c)
☐ ☐ ☐ ☐ ☐ ☐

Fruit – 4-6 servings per day; (serving= ½ c.)
☐ ☐ ☐ ☐ ☐ ☐

Milk & Milk Products – 2-3 servings (serving = 8 oz)
☐ ☐ ☐

Meat, Chicken, Fish – 6 servings (1 serving =1oz)
☐ ☐ ☐ ☐ ☐ ☐

Nuts, seeds, and legumes -- 4–5 per week
☐ ☐ ☐ ☐ ☐ ☐

Fats and oils – 2-3 per day
☐ ☐ ☐

Sweets and sugar – 5 servings or less per week
☐ ☐ ☐ ☐ ☐

How did you do today? √

A great day ☐ **Mostly followed DASH**☐ **I'll do better tomorrow** ☐

Your thoughts and feelings about dieting so far:

____

____

____

DAY **14**

Date: ____________

Time	Food	Comments

6-8 8 oz. glasses of water √ ☐ ☐ ☐ ☐ ☐ ☐ ☐ ☐

Exercise? ☐ **Yes** ☐ **No** _________ **minutes**

Exercise/Activity:

____

____

The Daily DASH Diet
2000 Calorie Plan (reduce or add food as needed)
Sodium Goal: 2300 mg/day or 1500 mg/day

Grains – 4-6 servings per day; try for whole grains
☐ ☐ ☐ ☐ ☐ ☐

Vegetables – 4-6 servings per day; (serving = ½ c)
☐ ☐ ☐ ☐ ☐ ☐

Fruit – 4-6 servings per day; (serving= ½ c.)
☐ ☐ ☐ ☐ ☐ ☐

Milk & Milk Products – 2-3 servings (serving = 8 oz)
☐ ☐ ☐

Meat, Chicken, Fish – 6 servings (1 serving =1oz)
☐ ☐ ☐ ☐ ☐ ☐

Nuts, seeds, and legumes -- 4–5 per week
☐ ☐ ☐ ☐ ☐ ☐

Fats and oils – 2-3 per day
☐ ☐ ☐

Sweets and sugar – 5 servings or less per week
☐ ☐ ☐ ☐ ☐

How did you do today? √

A great day ☐ **Mostly followed DASH**☐ **I'll do better tomorrow** ☐

Your thoughts and feelings about dieting so far:

____

____

____

DAY 15 **Date: __________**

Time	Food	Comments

6-8 8 oz. glasses of water √ ☐ ☐ ☐ ☐ ☐ ☐ ☐ ☐

Exercise? ☐ **Yes** ☐ **No** _________ **minutes**

Exercise/Activity:

____

____

The Daily DASH Diet

2000 Calorie Plan (reduce or add food as needed)

Sodium Goal: 2300 mg/day or 1500 mg/day

Grains – 4-6 servings per day; try for whole grains

☐ ☐ ☐ ☐ ☐ ☐

Vegetables – 4-6 servings per day; (serving = ½ c)

☐ ☐ ☐ ☐ ☐ ☐

Fruit – 4-6 servings per day; (serving= ½ c.)

☐ ☐ ☐ ☐ ☐ ☐

Milk & Milk Products – 2-3 servings (serving = 8 oz)

☐ ☐ ☐

Meat, Chicken, Fish – 6 servings (1 serving =1oz)

☐ ☐ ☐ ☐ ☐ ☐

Nuts, seeds, and legumes -- 4–5 per week

☐ ☐ ☐ ☐ ☐ ☐

Fats and oils – 2-3 per day

☐ ☐ ☐

Sweets and sugar – 5 servings or less per week

☐ ☐ ☐ ☐ ☐

How did you do today? √

A great day ☐ **Mostly followed DASH**☐ **I'll do better tomorrow** ☐

Your thoughts and feelings about dieting so far:

____

____

____

DAY 16 Date: ___________

Time	Food	Comments

6-8 8 oz. glasses of water √ ☐ ☐ ☐ ☐ ☐ ☐ ☐ ☐

Exercise? ☐ **Yes** ☐ **No** _________ **minutes**

Exercise/Activity:

____

____

The Daily DASH Diet
2000 Calorie Plan (reduce or add food as needed)
Sodium Goal: 2300 mg/day or 1500 mg/day

Grains – 4-6 servings per day; try for whole grains
☐ ☐ ☐ ☐ ☐ ☐

Vegetables – 4-6 servings per day; (serving = ½ c)
☐ ☐ ☐ ☐ ☐ ☐

Fruit – 4-6 servings per day; (serving= ½ c.)
☐ ☐ ☐ ☐ ☐ ☐

Milk & Milk Products – 2-3 servings (serving = 8 oz)
☐ ☐ ☐

Meat, Chicken, Fish – 6 servings (1 serving =1oz)
☐ ☐ ☐ ☐ ☐ ☐

Nuts, seeds, and legumes -- 4–5 per week
☐ ☐ ☐ ☐ ☐ ☐

Fats and oils – 2-3 per day
☐ ☐ ☐

Sweets and sugar – 5 servings or less per week
☐ ☐ ☐ ☐ ☐

How did you do today? √

A great day ☐ **Mostly followed DASH**☐ **I'll do better tomorrow** ☐

Your thoughts and feelings about dieting so far:

____

____

____

DAY 17 **Date: ___________**

Time	Food	Comments

6-8 8 oz. glasses of water √ ☐ ☐ ☐ ☐ ☐ ☐ ☐ ☐

Exercise? ☐ **Yes** ☐ **No** _________ **minutes**

Exercise/Activity:

____

____

The Daily DASH Diet
2000 Calorie Plan (reduce or add food as needed)
Sodium Goal: 2300 mg/day or 1500 mg/day

Grains – 4-6 servings per day; try for whole grains
☐ ☐ ☐ ☐ ☐ ☐

Vegetables – 4-6 servings per day; (serving = ½ c)
☐ ☐ ☐ ☐ ☐ ☐

Fruit – 4-6 servings per day; (serving= ½ c.)
☐ ☐ ☐ ☐ ☐ ☐

Milk & Milk Products – 2-3 servings (serving = 8 oz)
☐ ☐ ☐

Meat, Chicken, Fish – 6 servings (1 serving =1oz)
☐ ☐ ☐ ☐ ☐ ☐

Nuts, seeds, and legumes -- 4–5 per week
☐ ☐ ☐ ☐ ☐ ☐

Fats and oils – 2-3 per day
☐ ☐ ☐

Sweets and sugar – 5 servings or less per week
☐ ☐ ☐ ☐ ☐

How did you do today? √

A great day ☐ **Mostly followed DASH**☐ **I'll do better tomorrow** ☐

Your thoughts and feelings about dieting so far:

____

____

____

DAY 18 **Date: ____________**

Time	Food	Comments

6-8 8 oz. glasses of water √ ☐ ☐ ☐ ☐ ☐ ☐ ☐ ☐

Exercise? ☐ **Yes** ☐ **No** _________ **minutes**

Exercise/Activity:

____

____

The Daily DASH Diet
2000 Calorie Plan (reduce or add food as needed)
Sodium Goal: 2300 mg/day or 1500 mg/day

Grains – 4-6 servings per day; try for whole grains
☐ ☐ ☐ ☐ ☐ ☐

Vegetables – 4-6 servings per day; (serving = ½ c)
☐ ☐ ☐ ☐ ☐ ☐

Fruit – 4-6 servings per day; (serving= ½ c.)
☐ ☐ ☐ ☐ ☐ ☐

Milk & Milk Products – 2-3 servings (serving = 8 oz)
☐ ☐ ☐

Meat, Chicken, Fish – 6 servings (1 serving =1oz)
☐ ☐ ☐ ☐ ☐ ☐

Nuts, seeds, and legumes -- 4–5 per week
☐ ☐ ☐ ☐ ☐ ☐

Fats and oils – 2-3 per day
☐ ☐ ☐

Sweets and sugar – 5 servings or less per week
☐ ☐ ☐ ☐ ☐

How did you do today? √

A great day ☐ **Mostly followed DASH**☐ **I'll do better tomorrow** ☐

Your thoughts and feelings about dieting so far:

____

____

____

DAY 19

Date: ___________

Time	Food	Comments

6-8 8 oz. glasses of water √ ☐ ☐ ☐ ☐ ☐ ☐ ☐ ☐

Exercise? ☐ **Yes** ☐ **No** _________ **minutes**

Exercise/Activity:

____

____

The Daily DASH Diet
2000 Calorie Plan (reduce or add food as needed)
Sodium Goal: 2300 mg/day or 1500 mg/day

Grains – 4-6 servings per day; try for whole grains
☐ ☐ ☐ ☐ ☐ ☐

Vegetables – 4-6 servings per day; (serving = ½ c)
☐ ☐ ☐ ☐ ☐ ☐

Fruit – 4-6 servings per day; (serving= ½ c.)
☐ ☐ ☐ ☐ ☐ ☐

Milk & Milk Products – 2-3 servings (serving = 8 oz)
☐ ☐ ☐

Meat, Chicken, Fish – 6 servings (1 serving =1oz)
☐ ☐ ☐ ☐ ☐ ☐

Nuts, seeds, and legumes -- 4–5 per week
☐ ☐ ☐ ☐ ☐ ☐

Fats and oils – 2-3 per day
☐ ☐ ☐

Sweets and sugar – 5 servings or less per week
☐ ☐ ☐ ☐ ☐

How did you do today? √

A great day ☐ **Mostly followed DASH**☐ **I'll do better tomorrow** ☐

Your thoughts and feelings about dieting so far:

____

____

____

DAY 20 Date: ____________

Time	Food	Comments

6-8 8 oz. glasses of water √ ☐ ☐ ☐ ☐ ☐ ☐ ☐ ☐

Exercise? ☐ **Yes** ☐ **No** _________ **minutes**

Exercise/Activity:

____

____

The Daily DASH Diet
2000 Calorie Plan (reduce or add food as needed)
Sodium Goal: 2300 mg/day or 1500 mg/day

Grains – 4-6 servings per day; try for whole grains
☐ ☐ ☐ ☐ ☐ ☐

Vegetables – 4-6 servings per day; (serving = ½ c)
☐ ☐ ☐ ☐ ☐ ☐

Fruit – 4-6 servings per day; (serving= ½ c.)
☐ ☐ ☐ ☐ ☐ ☐

Milk & Milk Products – 2-3 servings (serving = 8 oz)
☐ ☐ ☐

Meat, Chicken, Fish – 6 servings (1 serving =1oz)
☐ ☐ ☐ ☐ ☐ ☐

Nuts, seeds, and legumes -- 4–5 per week
☐ ☐ ☐ ☐ ☐ ☐

Fats and oils – 2-3 per day
☐ ☐ ☐

Sweets and sugar – 5 servings or less per week
☐ ☐ ☐ ☐ ☐

How did you do today? √

A great day ☐ **Mostly followed DASH**☐ **I'll do better tomorrow** ☐

Your thoughts and feelings about dieting so far:

____

____

____

DAY 21 Date: ___________

Time	Food	Comments

6-8 8 oz. glasses of water √ ☐ ☐ ☐ ☐ ☐ ☐ ☐ ☐

Exercise? ☐ **Yes** ☐ **No** _________ **minutes**

Exercise/Activity:

____

____

The Daily DASH Diet
2000 Calorie Plan (reduce or add food as needed)
Sodium Goal: 2300 mg/day or 1500 mg/day

Grains – 4-6 servings per day; try for whole grains
☐ ☐ ☐ ☐ ☐ ☐

Vegetables – 4-6 servings per day; (serving = ½ c)
☐ ☐ ☐ ☐ ☐ ☐

Fruit – 4-6 servings per day; (serving= ½ c.)
☐ ☐ ☐ ☐ ☐ ☐

Milk & Milk Products – 2-3 servings (serving = 8 oz)
☐ ☐ ☐

Meat, Chicken, Fish – 6 servings (1 serving =1oz)
☐ ☐ ☐ ☐ ☐ ☐

Nuts, seeds, and legumes -- 4–5 per week
☐ ☐ ☐ ☐ ☐ ☐

Fats and oils – 2-3 per day
☐ ☐ ☐

Sweets and sugar – 5 servings or less per week
☐ ☐ ☐ ☐ ☐

How did you do today? √

A great day ☐ **Mostly followed DASH**☐ **I'll do better tomorrow** ☐

Your thoughts and feelings about dieting so far:

____

____

____

DAY **22** Date: ____________

Time	Food	Comments

6-8 8 oz. glasses of water √ ☐ ☐ ☐ ☐ ☐ ☐ ☐ ☐

Exercise? ☐ **Yes** ☐ **No** ________ **minutes**

Exercise/Activity:

____

____

The Daily DASH Diet
2000 Calorie Plan (reduce or add food as needed)
Sodium Goal: 2300 mg/day or 1500 mg/day

Grains – 4-6 servings per day; try for whole grains
☐ ☐ ☐ ☐ ☐ ☐

Vegetables – 4-6 servings per day; (serving = ½ c)
☐ ☐ ☐ ☐ ☐ ☐

Fruit – 4-6 servings per day; (serving= ½ c.)
☐ ☐ ☐ ☐ ☐ ☐

Milk & Milk Products – 2-3 servings (serving = 8 oz)
☐ ☐ ☐

Meat, Chicken, Fish – 6 servings (1 serving =1oz)
☐ ☐ ☐ ☐ ☐ ☐

Nuts, seeds, and legumes -- 4–5 per week
☐ ☐ ☐ ☐ ☐ ☐

Fats and oils – 2-3 per day
☐ ☐ ☐

Sweets and sugar – 5 servings or less per week
☐ ☐ ☐ ☐ ☐

How did you do today? √

A great day ☐ **Mostly followed DASH**☐ **I'll do better tomorrow** ☐

Your thoughts and feelings about dieting so far:

____

____

____

DAY **23** Date: ___________

Time	Food	Comments

6-8 8 oz. glasses of water √ ☐ ☐ ☐ ☐ ☐ ☐ ☐ ☐

Exercise? ☐ **Yes** ☐ **No** _________ **minutes**

Exercise/Activity:

____

____

The Daily DASH Diet
2000 Calorie Plan (reduce or add food as needed)
Sodium Goal: 2300 mg/day or 1500 mg/day

Grains – 4-6 servings per day; try for whole grains
☐ ☐ ☐ ☐ ☐ ☐

Vegetables – 4-6 servings per day; (serving = ½ c)
☐ ☐ ☐ ☐ ☐ ☐

Fruit – 4-6 servings per day; (serving= ½ c.)
☐ ☐ ☐ ☐ ☐ ☐

Milk & Milk Products – 2-3 servings (serving = 8 oz)
☐ ☐ ☐

Meat, Chicken, Fish – 6 servings (1 serving =1oz)
☐ ☐ ☐ ☐ ☐ ☐

Nuts, seeds, and legumes -- 4–5 per week
☐ ☐ ☐ ☐ ☐ ☐

Fats and oils – 2-3 per day
☐ ☐ ☐

Sweets and sugar – 5 servings or less per week
☐ ☐ ☐ ☐ ☐

How did you do today? √

A great day ☐ **Mostly followed DASH**☐ **I'll do better tomorrow** ☐

Your thoughts and feelings about dieting so far:

____

____

____

DAY **24**

Date: ___________

Time	Food	Comments

6-8 8 oz. glasses of water √ ☐ ☐ ☐ ☐ ☐ ☐ ☐ ☐

Exercise? ☐ Yes ☐ No _________ minutes

Exercise/Activity:

____

____

The Daily DASH Diet
2000 Calorie Plan (reduce or add food as needed)
Sodium Goal: 2300 mg/day or 1500 mg/day

Grains – 4-6 servings per day; try for whole grains
☐ ☐ ☐ ☐ ☐ ☐

Vegetables – 4-6 servings per day; (serving = ½ c)
☐ ☐ ☐ ☐ ☐ ☐

Fruit – 4-6 servings per day; (serving= ½ c.)
☐ ☐ ☐ ☐ ☐ ☐

Milk & Milk Products – 2-3 servings (serving = 8 oz)
☐ ☐ ☐

Meat, Chicken, Fish – 6 servings (1 serving =1oz)
☐ ☐ ☐ ☐ ☐ ☐

Nuts, seeds, and legumes -- 4–5 per week
☐ ☐ ☐ ☐ ☐ ☐

Fats and oils – 2-3 per day
☐ ☐ ☐

Sweets and sugar – 5 servings or less per week
☐ ☐ ☐ ☐ ☐

How did you do today? √

A great day ☐ Mostly followed DASH☐ I'll do better tomorrow ☐

Your thoughts and feelings about dieting so far:

____

____

____

DAY 25 **Date: ____________**

Time	Food	Comments

6-8 8 oz. glasses of water √ ☐ ☐ ☐ ☐ ☐ ☐ ☐ ☐

Exercise? ☐ **Yes** ☐ **No** _________ **minutes**

Exercise/Activity:

____

____

The Daily DASH Diet

2000 Calorie Plan (reduce or add food as needed)

Sodium Goal: 2300 mg/day or 1500 mg/day

Grains – 4-6 servings per day; try for whole grains
☐ ☐ ☐ ☐ ☐ ☐

Vegetables – 4-6 servings per day; (serving = ½ c)
☐ ☐ ☐ ☐ ☐ ☐

Fruit – 4-6 servings per day; (serving= ½ c.)
☐ ☐ ☐ ☐ ☐ ☐

Milk & Milk Products – 2-3 servings (serving = 8 oz)
☐ ☐ ☐

Meat, Chicken, Fish – 6 servings (1 serving =1oz)
☐ ☐ ☐ ☐ ☐ ☐

Nuts, seeds, and legumes -- 4–5 per week
☐ ☐ ☐ ☐ ☐ ☐

Fats and oils – 2-3 per day
☐ ☐ ☐

Sweets and sugar – 5 servings or less per week
☐ ☐ ☐ ☐ ☐

How did you do today? √

A great day ☐ **Mostly followed DASH**☐ **I'll do better tomorrow** ☐

Your thoughts and feelings about dieting so far:

____

____

____

DAY **26** Date: ____________

Time	Food	Comments

6-8 8 oz. glasses of water √ ☐ ☐ ☐ ☐ ☐ ☐ ☐ ☐

Exercise? ☐ **Yes** ☐ **No** _________ **minutes**

Exercise/Activity:

____

____

The Daily DASH Diet
2000 Calorie Plan (reduce or add food as needed)
Sodium Goal: 2300 mg/day or 1500 mg/day

Grains – 4-6 servings per day; try for whole grains
☐ ☐ ☐ ☐ ☐ ☐

Vegetables – 4-6 servings per day; (serving = ½ c)
☐ ☐ ☐ ☐ ☐ ☐

Fruit – 4-6 servings per day; (serving= ½ c.)
☐ ☐ ☐ ☐ ☐ ☐

Milk & Milk Products – 2-3 servings (serving = 8 oz)
☐ ☐ ☐

Meat, Chicken, Fish – 6 servings (1 serving =1oz)
☐ ☐ ☐ ☐ ☐ ☐

Nuts, seeds, and legumes -- 4–5 per week
☐ ☐ ☐ ☐ ☐ ☐

Fats and oils – 2-3 per day
☐ ☐ ☐

Sweets and sugar – 5 servings or less per week
☐ ☐ ☐ ☐ ☐

How did you do today? √

A great day ☐ **Mostly followed DASH**☐ **I'll do better tomorrow** ☐

Your thoughts and feelings about dieting so far:

____

____

____

DAY 27 **Date: ____________**

Time	Food	Comments

6-8 8 oz. glasses of water √ ☐ ☐ ☐ ☐ ☐ ☐ ☐ ☐

Exercise? ☐ **Yes** ☐ **No** ________ **minutes**

Exercise/Activity:

____

____

The Daily DASH Diet
2000 Calorie Plan (reduce or add food as needed)
Sodium Goal: 2300 mg/day or 1500 mg/day

Grains – 4-6 servings per day; try for whole grains
☐ ☐ ☐ ☐ ☐ ☐

Vegetables – 4-6 servings per day; (serving = ½ c)
☐ ☐ ☐ ☐ ☐ ☐

Fruit – 4-6 servings per day; (serving= ½ c.)
☐ ☐ ☐ ☐ ☐ ☐

Milk & Milk Products – 2-3 servings (serving = 8 oz)
☐ ☐ ☐

Meat, Chicken, Fish – 6 servings (1 serving =1oz)
☐ ☐ ☐ ☐ ☐ ☐

Nuts, seeds, and legumes -- 4–5 per week
☐ ☐ ☐ ☐ ☐ ☐

Fats and oils – 2-3 per day
☐ ☐ ☐

Sweets and sugar – 5 servings or less per week
☐ ☐ ☐ ☐ ☐

How did you do today? √

A great day ☐ **Mostly followed DASH**☐ **I'll do better tomorrow** ☐

Your thoughts and feelings about dieting so far:

____

____

____

DAY **28** Date: ___________

Time	Food	Comments

6-8 8 oz. glasses of water √ ☐ ☐ ☐ ☐ ☐ ☐ ☐ ☐

Exercise? ▫ **Yes** ▫ **No** ________ **minutes**

Exercise/Activity:

____

____

The Daily DASH Diet
2000 Calorie Plan (reduce or add food as needed)
Sodium Goal: 2300 mg/day or 1500 mg/day

Grains – 4-6 servings per day; try for whole grains
☐ ☐ ☐ ☐ ☐ ☐
Vegetables – 4-6 servings per day; (serving = ½ c)
☐ ☐ ☐ ☐ ☐ ☐
Fruit – 4-6 servings per day; (serving= ½ c.)
☐ ☐ ☐ ☐ ☐ ☐
Milk & Milk Products – 2-3 servings (serving = 8 oz)
☐ ☐ ☐
Meat, Chicken, Fish – 6 servings (1 serving =1oz)
☐ ☐ ☐ ☐ ☐ ☐
Nuts, seeds, and legumes -- 4–5 per week
☐ ☐ ☐ ☐ ☐ ☐
Fats and oils – 2-3 per day
☐ ☐ ☐
Sweets and sugar – 5 servings or less per week
☐ ☐ ☐ ☐ ☐

How did you do today? √

A great day ☐ **Mostly followed DASH**☐ **I'll do better tomorrow** ☐

Your thoughts and feelings about dieting so far:

____

____

____

DAY **29**

Date: ____________

Time	Food	Comments

6-8 8 oz. glasses of water √ ☐ ☐ ☐ ☐ ☐ ☐ ☐ ☐

Exercise? ☐ **Yes** ☐ **No** _________ **minutes**

Exercise/Activity:

____

____

The Daily DASH Diet
2000 Calorie Plan (reduce or add food as needed)
Sodium Goal: 2300 mg/day or 1500 mg/day

Grains – 4-6 servings per day; try for whole grains
☐ ☐ ☐ ☐ ☐ ☐

Vegetables – 4-6 servings per day; (serving = ½ c)
☐ ☐ ☐ ☐ ☐ ☐

Fruit – 4-6 servings per day; (serving= ½ c.)
☐ ☐ ☐ ☐ ☐ ☐

Milk & Milk Products – 2-3 servings (serving = 8 oz)
☐ ☐ ☐

Meat, Chicken, Fish – 6 servings (1 serving =1oz)
☐ ☐ ☐ ☐ ☐ ☐

Nuts, seeds, and legumes -- 4–5 per week
☐ ☐ ☐ ☐ ☐ ☐

Fats and oils – 2-3 per day
☐ ☐ ☐

Sweets and sugar – 5 servings or less per week
☐ ☐ ☐ ☐ ☐

How did you do today? √

A great day ☐ **Mostly followed DASH**☐ **I'll do better tomorrow** ☐

Your thoughts and feelings about dieting so far:

____

____

____

DAY **30**

Date: ____________

Time	Food	Comments

6-8 8 oz. glasses of water √ ☐ ☐ ☐ ☐ ☐ ☐ ☐ ☐

Exercise? ☐ **Yes** ☐ **No** _________ **minutes**

Exercise/Activity:

____

____

The Daily DASH Diet
2000 Calorie Plan (reduce or add food as needed)
Sodium Goal: 2300 mg/day or 1500 mg/day

Grains – 4-6 servings per day; try for whole grains
☐ ☐ ☐ ☐ ☐ ☐

Vegetables – 4-6 servings per day; (serving = ½ c)
☐ ☐ ☐ ☐ ☐ ☐

Fruit – 4-6 servings per day; (serving= ½ c.)
☐ ☐ ☐ ☐ ☐ ☐

Milk & Milk Products – 2-3 servings (serving = 8 oz)
☐ ☐ ☐

Meat, Chicken, Fish – 6 servings (1 serving =1oz)
☐ ☐ ☐ ☐ ☐ ☐

Nuts, seeds, and legumes -- 4–5 per week
☐ ☐ ☐ ☐ ☐ ☐

Fats and oils – 2-3 per day
☐ ☐ ☐

Sweets and sugar – 5 servings or less per week
☐ ☐ ☐ ☐ ☐

How did you do today? √

A great day ☐ **Mostly followed DASH**☐ **I'll do better tomorrow** ☐

Your thoughts and feelings about dieting so far:

____

____

____

DAY 31 Date: ___________

Time	Food	Comments

6-8 8 oz. glasses of water √ ☐ ☐ ☐ ☐ ☐ ☐ ☐ ☐

Exercise? ☐ **Yes** ☐ **No** _________ **minutes**

Exercise/Activity:

____

____

The Daily DASH Diet
2000 Calorie Plan (reduce or add food as needed)
Sodium Goal: 2300 mg/day or 1500 mg/day

Grains – 4-6 servings per day; try for whole grains
☐ ☐ ☐ ☐ ☐ ☐

Vegetables – 4-6 servings per day; (serving = ½ c)
☐ ☐ ☐ ☐ ☐ ☐

Fruit – 4-6 servings per day; (serving= ½ c.)
☐ ☐ ☐ ☐ ☐ ☐

Milk & Milk Products – 2-3 servings (serving = 8 oz)
☐ ☐ ☐

Meat, Chicken, Fish – 6 servings (1 serving =1oz)
☐ ☐ ☐ ☐ ☐ ☐

Nuts, seeds, and legumes -- 4–5 per week
☐ ☐ ☐ ☐ ☐ ☐

Fats and oils – 2-3 per day
☐ ☐ ☐

Sweets and sugar – 5 servings or less per week
☐ ☐ ☐ ☐ ☐

How did you do today? √

A great day ☐ **Mostly followed DASH**☐ **I'll do better tomorrow** ☐

Your thoughts and feelings about dieting so far:

____

____

____

DAY 32 **Date: ___________**

Time	Food	Comments

6-8 8 oz. glasses of water √ ☐ ☐ ☐ ☐ ☐ ☐ ☐ ☐

Exercise? ☐ **Yes** ☐ **No** _________ **minutes**

Exercise/Activity:

____

____

The Daily DASH Diet
2000 Calorie Plan (reduce or add food as needed)
Sodium Goal: 2300 mg/day or 1500 mg/day

Grains – 4-6 servings per day; try for whole grains
☐ ☐ ☐ ☐ ☐ ☐

Vegetables – 4-6 servings per day; (serving = ½ c)
☐ ☐ ☐ ☐ ☐ ☐

Fruit – 4-6 servings per day; (serving= ½ c.)
☐ ☐ ☐ ☐ ☐ ☐

Milk & Milk Products – 2-3 servings (serving = 8 oz)
☐ ☐ ☐

Meat, Chicken, Fish – 6 servings (1 serving =1oz)
☐ ☐ ☐ ☐ ☐ ☐

Nuts, seeds, and legumes -- 4–5 per week
☐ ☐ ☐ ☐ ☐ ☐

Fats and oils – 2-3 per day
☐ ☐ ☐

Sweets and sugar – 5 servings or less per week
☐ ☐ ☐ ☐ ☐

How did you do today? √

A great day ☐ **Mostly followed DASH**☐ **I'll do better tomorrow** ☐

Your thoughts and feelings about dieting so far:

____

____

____

DAY 33 **Date: ____________**

Time	Food	Comments

6-8 8 oz. glasses of water √ ☐ ☐ ☐ ☐ ☐ ☐ ☐ ☐

Exercise? ☐ **Yes** ☐ **No** _________ **minutes**

Exercise/Activity:

____

____

The Daily DASH Diet
2000 Calorie Plan (reduce or add food as needed)
Sodium Goal: 2300 mg/day or 1500 mg/day

Grains – 4-6 servings per day; try for whole grains
☐ ☐ ☐ ☐ ☐ ☐

Vegetables – 4-6 servings per day; (serving = ½ c)
☐ ☐ ☐ ☐ ☐ ☐

Fruit – 4-6 servings per day; (serving= ½ c.)
☐ ☐ ☐ ☐ ☐ ☐

Milk & Milk Products – 2-3 servings (serving = 8 oz)
☐ ☐ ☐

Meat, Chicken, Fish – 6 servings (1 serving =1oz)
☐ ☐ ☐ ☐ ☐ ☐

Nuts, seeds, and legumes -- 4–5 per week
☐ ☐ ☐ ☐ ☐ ☐

Fats and oils – 2-3 per day
☐ ☐ ☐

Sweets and sugar – 5 servings or less per week
☐ ☐ ☐ ☐ ☐

How did you do today? √

A great day ☐ **Mostly followed DASH** ☐ **I'll do better tomorrow** ☐

Your thoughts and feelings about dieting so far:

____

____

____

DAY **34** Date: ____________

Time	Food	Comments

6-8 8 oz. glasses of water √ ☐ ☐ ☐ ☐ ☐ ☐ ☐ ☐

Exercise? ☐ **Yes** ☐ **No** _________ **minutes**

Exercise/Activity:

____

____

The Daily DASH Diet
2000 Calorie Plan (reduce or add food as needed)
Sodium Goal: 2300 mg/day or 1500 mg/day

Grains – 4-6 servings per day; try for whole grains
☐ ☐ ☐ ☐ ☐ ☐

Vegetables – 4-6 servings per day; (serving = ½ c)
☐ ☐ ☐ ☐ ☐ ☐

Fruit – 4-6 servings per day; (serving= ½ c.)
☐ ☐ ☐ ☐ ☐ ☐

Milk & Milk Products – 2-3 servings (serving = 8 oz)
☐ ☐ ☐

Meat, Chicken, Fish – 6 servings (1 serving =1oz)
☐ ☐ ☐ ☐ ☐ ☐

Nuts, seeds, and legumes -- 4–5 per week
☐ ☐ ☐ ☐ ☐ ☐

Fats and oils – 2-3 per day
☐ ☐ ☐

Sweets and sugar – 5 servings or less per week
☐ ☐ ☐ ☐ ☐

How did you do today? √

A great day ☐ **Mostly followed DASH**☐ **I'll do better tomorrow** ☐

Your thoughts and feelings about dieting so far:

____

____

____

DAY 35 **Date: ____________**

Time	Food	Comments

6-8 8 oz. glasses of water √ ☐ ☐ ☐ ☐ ☐ ☐ ☐ ☐

Exercise? ☐ **Yes** ☐ **No** _________ **minutes**

Exercise/Activity:

____

____

The Daily DASH Diet
2000 Calorie Plan (reduce or add food as needed)
Sodium Goal: 2300 mg/day or 1500 mg/day

Grains – 4-6 servings per day; try for whole grains
☐ ☐ ☐ ☐ ☐ ☐

Vegetables – 4-6 servings per day; (serving = ½ c)
☐ ☐ ☐ ☐ ☐ ☐

Fruit – 4-6 servings per day; (serving= ½ c.)
☐ ☐ ☐ ☐ ☐ ☐

Milk & Milk Products – 2-3 servings (serving = 8 oz)
☐ ☐ ☐

Meat, Chicken, Fish – 6 servings (1 serving =1oz)
☐ ☐ ☐ ☐ ☐ ☐

Nuts, seeds, and legumes -- 4–5 per week
☐ ☐ ☐ ☐ ☐ ☐

Fats and oils – 2-3 per day
☐ ☐ ☐

Sweets and sugar – 5 servings or less per week
☐ ☐ ☐ ☐ ☐

How did you do today? √

A great day ☐ **Mostly followed DASH**☐ **I'll do better tomorrow** ☐

Your thoughts and feelings about dieting so far:

____

____

____

DAY **36** Date: ___________

Time	Food	Comments

6-8 8 oz. glasses of water √ ☐ ☐ ☐ ☐ ☐ ☐ ☐ ☐

Exercise? ☐ **Yes** ☐ **No** _________ **minutes**

Exercise/Activity:

____

____

The Daily DASH Diet
2000 Calorie Plan (reduce or add food as needed)
Sodium Goal: 2300 mg/day or 1500 mg/day

Grains – 4-6 servings per day; try for whole grains
☐ ☐ ☐ ☐ ☐ ☐
Vegetables – 4-6 servings per day; (serving = ½ c)
☐ ☐ ☐ ☐ ☐ ☐
Fruit – 4-6 servings per day; (serving= ½ c.)
☐ ☐ ☐ ☐ ☐ ☐
Milk & Milk Products – 2-3 servings (serving = 8 oz)
☐ ☐ ☐
Meat, Chicken, Fish – 6 servings (1 serving =1oz)
☐ ☐ ☐ ☐ ☐ ☐
Nuts, seeds, and legumes -- 4–5 per week
☐ ☐ ☐ ☐ ☐ ☐
Fats and oils – 2-3 per day
☐ ☐ ☐
Sweets and sugar – 5 servings or less per week
☐ ☐ ☐ ☐ ☐

How did you do today? √

A great day ☐ **Mostly followed DASH**☐ **I'll do better tomorrow** ☐

Your thoughts and feelings about dieting so far:

____

____

____

DAY 37 Date: ___________

Time	Food	Comments

6-8 8 oz. glasses of water √ ☐ ☐ ☐ ☐ ☐ ☐ ☐ ☐

Exercise? ☐ **Yes** ☐ **No** _________ **minutes**

Exercise/Activity:

____

____

The Daily DASH Diet

2000 Calorie Plan (reduce or add food as needed)

Sodium Goal: 2300 mg/day or 1500 mg/day

Grains – 4-6 servings per day; try for whole grains

☐ ☐ ☐ ☐ ☐ ☐

Vegetables – 4-6 servings per day; (serving = ½ c)

☐ ☐ ☐ ☐ ☐ ☐

Fruit – 4-6 servings per day; (serving= ½ c.)

☐ ☐ ☐ ☐ ☐ ☐

Milk & Milk Products – 2-3 servings (serving = 8 oz)

☐ ☐ ☐

Meat, Chicken, Fish – 6 servings (1 serving =1oz)

☐ ☐ ☐ ☐ ☐ ☐

Nuts, seeds, and legumes -- 4–5 per week

☐ ☐ ☐ ☐ ☐ ☐

Fats and oils – 2-3 per day

☐ ☐ ☐

Sweets and sugar – 5 servings or less per week

☐ ☐ ☐ ☐ ☐

How did you do today? √

A great day ☐ **Mostly followed DASH**☐ **I'll do better tomorrow** ☐

Your thoughts and feelings about dieting so far:

____

____

____

DAY **38** Date: ___________

Time	Food	Comments

6-8 8 oz. glasses of water √ ☐ ☐ ☐ ☐ ☐ ☐ ☐ ☐

Exercise? ☐ **Yes** ☐ **No** _________ **minutes**

Exercise/Activity:

____

____

The Daily DASH Diet
2000 Calorie Plan (reduce or add food as needed)
Sodium Goal: 2300 mg/day or 1500 mg/day

Grains – 4-6 servings per day; try for whole grains
☐ ☐ ☐ ☐ ☐ ☐

Vegetables – 4-6 servings per day; (serving = ½ c)
☐ ☐ ☐ ☐ ☐ ☐

Fruit – 4-6 servings per day; (serving= ½ c.)
☐ ☐ ☐ ☐ ☐ ☐

Milk & Milk Products – 2-3 servings (serving = 8 oz)
☐ ☐ ☐

Meat, Chicken, Fish – 6 servings (1 serving =1oz)
☐ ☐ ☐ ☐ ☐ ☐

Nuts, seeds, and legumes -- 4–5 per week
☐ ☐ ☐ ☐ ☐ ☐

Fats and oils – 2-3 per day
☐ ☐ ☐

Sweets and sugar – 5 servings or less per week
☐ ☐ ☐ ☐ ☐

How did you do today? √

A great day ☐ **Mostly followed DASH**☐ **I'll do better tomorrow** ☐

Your thoughts and feelings about dieting so far:

____

____

____

DAY 39 **Date:** ____________

Time	Food	Comments

6-8 8 oz. glasses of water √ ☐ ☐ ☐ ☐ ☐ ☐ ☐ ☐

Exercise? ☐ **Yes** ☐ **No** _________ **minutes**

Exercise/Activity:

____

____

The Daily DASH Diet
2000 Calorie Plan (reduce or add food as needed)
Sodium Goal: 2300 mg/day or 1500 mg/day

Grains – 4-6 servings per day; try for whole grains
☐ ☐ ☐ ☐ ☐ ☐

Vegetables – 4-6 servings per day; (serving = ½ c)
☐ ☐ ☐ ☐ ☐ ☐

Fruit – 4-6 servings per day; (serving= ½ c.)
☐ ☐ ☐ ☐ ☐ ☐

Milk & Milk Products – 2-3 servings (serving = 8 oz)
☐ ☐ ☐

Meat, Chicken, Fish – 6 servings (1 serving =1oz)
☐ ☐ ☐ ☐ ☐ ☐

Nuts, seeds, and legumes -- 4–5 per week
☐ ☐ ☐ ☐ ☐ ☐

Fats and oils – 2-3 per day
☐ ☐ ☐

Sweets and sugar – 5 servings or less per week
☐ ☐ ☐ ☐ ☐

How did you do today? √

A great day ☐ **Mostly followed DASH**☐ **I'll do better tomorrow** ☐

Your thoughts and feelings about dieting so far:

____

____

____

DAY **40** Date: ___________

Time	Food	Comments

6-8 8 oz. glasses of water √ ☐ ☐ ☐ ☐ ☐ ☐ ☐ ☐

Exercise? ☐ **Yes** ☐ **No** _________ **minutes**

Exercise/Activity:

____

____

The Daily DASH Diet
2000 Calorie Plan (reduce or add food as needed)
Sodium Goal: 2300 mg/day or 1500 mg/day

Grains – 4-6 servings per day; try for whole grains
☐ ☐ ☐ ☐ ☐ ☐

Vegetables – 4-6 servings per day; (serving = ½ c)
☐ ☐ ☐ ☐ ☐ ☐

Fruit – 4-6 servings per day; (serving= ½ c.)
☐ ☐ ☐ ☐ ☐ ☐

Milk & Milk Products – 2-3 servings (serving = 8 oz)
☐ ☐ ☐

Meat, Chicken, Fish – 6 servings (1 serving =1oz)
☐ ☐ ☐ ☐ ☐ ☐

Nuts, seeds, and legumes -- 4–5 per week
☐ ☐ ☐ ☐ ☐ ☐

Fats and oils – 2-3 per day
☐ ☐ ☐

Sweets and sugar – 5 servings or less per week
☐ ☐ ☐ ☐ ☐

How did you do today? √

A great day ☐ **Mostly followed DASH**☐ **I'll do better tomorrow** ☐

Your thoughts and feelings about dieting so far:

____

____

____

DAY **41**

Date: ___________

Time	Food	Comments

6-8 8 oz. glasses of water √ ☐ ☐ ☐ ☐ ☐ ☐ ☐ ☐

Exercise? ☐ **Yes** ☐ **No** _________ **minutes**

Exercise/Activity:

____

____

The Daily DASH Diet
2000 Calorie Plan (reduce or add food as needed)
Sodium Goal: 2300 mg/day or 1500 mg/day

Grains – 4-6 servings per day; try for whole grains
☐ ☐ ☐ ☐ ☐ ☐

Vegetables – 4-6 servings per day; (serving = ½ c)
☐ ☐ ☐ ☐ ☐ ☐

Fruit – 4-6 servings per day; (serving= ½ c.)
☐ ☐ ☐ ☐ ☐ ☐

Milk & Milk Products – 2-3 servings (serving = 8 oz)
☐ ☐ ☐

Meat, Chicken, Fish – 6 servings (1 serving =1oz)
☐ ☐ ☐ ☐ ☐ ☐

Nuts, seeds, and legumes -- 4–5 per week
☐ ☐ ☐ ☐ ☐ ☐

Fats and oils – 2-3 per day
☐ ☐ ☐

Sweets and sugar – 5 servings or less per week
☐ ☐ ☐ ☐ ☐

How did you do today? √

A great day ☐ **Mostly followed DASH**☐ **I'll do better tomorrow** ☐

Your thoughts and feelings about dieting so far:

____

____

____

DAY **42** Date: ____________

Time	Food	Comments

6-8 8 oz. glasses of water √ ☐ ☐ ☐ ☐ ☐ ☐ ☐ ☐

Exercise? ☐ **Yes** ☐ **No** _________ **minutes**

Exercise/Activity:

____

____

The Daily DASH Diet
2000 Calorie Plan (reduce or add food as needed)
Sodium Goal: 2300 mg/day or 1500 mg/day

Grains – 4-6 servings per day; try for whole grains
☐ ☐ ☐ ☐ ☐ ☐

Vegetables – 4-6 servings per day; (serving = ½ c)
☐ ☐ ☐ ☐ ☐ ☐

Fruit – 4-6 servings per day; (serving= ½ c.)
☐ ☐ ☐ ☐ ☐ ☐

Milk & Milk Products – 2-3 servings (serving = 8 oz)
☐ ☐ ☐

Meat, Chicken, Fish – 6 servings (1 serving =1oz)
☐ ☐ ☐ ☐ ☐ ☐

Nuts, seeds, and legumes -- 4–5 per week
☐ ☐ ☐ ☐ ☐ ☐

Fats and oils – 2-3 per day
☐ ☐ ☐

Sweets and sugar – 5 servings or less per week
☐ ☐ ☐ ☐ ☐

How did you do today? √

A great day ☐ **Mostly followed DASH**☐ **I'll do better tomorrow** ☐

Your thoughts and feelings about dieting so far:

____

____

____

DAY 43

Date: ___________

Time	Food	Comments

6-8 8 oz. glasses of water √ ☐ ☐ ☐ ☐ ☐ ☐ ☐ ☐

Exercise? ☐ **Yes** ☐ **No** _________ **minutes**

Exercise/Activity:

____

____

The Daily DASH Diet
2000 Calorie Plan (reduce or add food as needed)
Sodium Goal: 2300 mg/day or 1500 mg/day

Grains – 4-6 servings per day; try for whole grains
☐ ☐ ☐ ☐ ☐ ☐

Vegetables – 4-6 servings per day; (serving = ½ c)
☐ ☐ ☐ ☐ ☐ ☐

Fruit – 4-6 servings per day; (serving= ½ c.)
☐ ☐ ☐ ☐ ☐ ☐

Milk & Milk Products – 2-3 servings (serving = 8 oz)
☐ ☐ ☐

Meat, Chicken, Fish – 6 servings (1 serving =1oz)
☐ ☐ ☐ ☐ ☐ ☐

Nuts, seeds, and legumes -- 4–5 per week
☐ ☐ ☐ ☐ ☐ ☐

Fats and oils – 2-3 per day
☐ ☐ ☐

Sweets and sugar – 5 servings or less per week
☐ ☐ ☐ ☐ ☐

How did you do today? √

A great day ☐ **Mostly followed DASH**☐ **I'll do better tomorrow** ☐

Your thoughts and feelings about dieting so far:

____

____

____

DAY **44**

Date: ____________

Time	Food	Comments

6-8 8 oz. glasses of water √ ☐ ☐ ☐ ☐ ☐ ☐ ☐ ☐

Exercise? ☐ **Yes** ☐ **No** _________ **minutes**

Exercise/Activity:

____

____

The Daily DASH Diet
2000 Calorie Plan (reduce or add food as needed)
Sodium Goal: 2300 mg/day or 1500 mg/day

Grains – 4-6 servings per day; try for whole grains
☐ ☐ ☐ ☐ ☐ ☐

Vegetables – 4-6 servings per day; (serving = ½ c)
☐ ☐ ☐ ☐ ☐ ☐

Fruit – 4-6 servings per day; (serving= ½ c.)
☐ ☐ ☐ ☐ ☐ ☐

Milk & Milk Products – 2-3 servings (serving = 8 oz)
☐ ☐ ☐

Meat, Chicken, Fish – 6 servings (1 serving =1oz)
☐ ☐ ☐ ☐ ☐ ☐

Nuts, seeds, and legumes -- 4–5 per week
☐ ☐ ☐ ☐ ☐ ☐

Fats and oils – 2-3 per day
☐ ☐ ☐

Sweets and sugar – 5 servings or less per week
☐ ☐ ☐ ☐ ☐

How did you do today? √

A great day ☐ **Mostly followed DASH**☐ **I'll do better tomorrow** ☐

Your thoughts and feelings about dieting so far:

____

____

____

DAY **45**

Date: ____________

Time	Food	Comments

6-8 8 oz. glasses of water √ ☐ ☐ ☐ ☐ ☐ ☐ ☐ ☐

Exercise? ☐ **Yes** ☐ **No** ________ **minutes**

Exercise/Activity:

____

____

The Daily DASH Diet
2000 Calorie Plan (reduce or add food as needed)
Sodium Goal: 2300 mg/day or 1500 mg/day

Grains – 4-6 servings per day; try for whole grains
☐ ☐ ☐ ☐ ☐ ☐

Vegetables – 4-6 servings per day; (serving = ½ c)
☐ ☐ ☐ ☐ ☐ ☐

Fruit – 4-6 servings per day; (serving= ½ c.)
☐ ☐ ☐ ☐ ☐ ☐

Milk & Milk Products – 2-3 servings (serving = 8 oz)
☐ ☐ ☐

Meat, Chicken, Fish – 6 servings (1 serving =1oz)
☐ ☐ ☐ ☐ ☐ ☐

Nuts, seeds, and legumes -- 4–5 per week
☐ ☐ ☐ ☐ ☐ ☐

Fats and oils – 2-3 per day
☐ ☐ ☐

Sweets and sugar – 5 servings or less per week
☐ ☐ ☐ ☐ ☐

How did you do today? √

A great day ☐ **Mostly followed DASH**☐ **I'll do better tomorrow** ☐

Your thoughts and feelings about dieting so far:

____

____

____

DAY **46**

Date: ___________

Time	Food	Comments

6-8 8 oz. glasses of water √ ☐ ☐ ☐ ☐ ☐ ☐ ☐ ☐

Exercise? ☐ Yes ☐ No _________ minutes

Exercise/Activity:

___

___

The Daily DASH Diet
2000 Calorie Plan (reduce or add food as needed)
Sodium Goal: 2300 mg/day or 1500 mg/day

Grains – 4-6 servings per day; try for whole grains
☐ ☐ ☐ ☐ ☐ ☐

Vegetables – 4-6 servings per day; (serving = ½ c)
☐ ☐ ☐ ☐ ☐ ☐

Fruit – 4-6 servings per day; (serving= ½ c.)
☐ ☐ ☐ ☐ ☐ ☐

Milk & Milk Products – 2-3 servings (serving = 8 oz)
☐ ☐ ☐

Meat, Chicken, Fish – 6 servings (1 serving =1oz)
☐ ☐ ☐ ☐ ☐ ☐

Nuts, seeds, and legumes -- 4–5 per week
☐ ☐ ☐ ☐ ☐ ☐

Fats and oils – 2-3 per day
☐ ☐ ☐

Sweets and sugar – 5 servings or less per week
☐ ☐ ☐ ☐ ☐

How did you do today? √

A great day ☐ Mostly followed DASH☐ I'll do better tomorrow ☐

Your thoughts and feelings about dieting so far:

___

___

___

DAY 47 **Date: ____________**

Time	Food	Comments

6-8 8 oz. glasses of water √ ☐ ☐ ☐ ☐ ☐ ☐ ☐ ☐

Exercise? ☐ **Yes** ☐ **No** _________ **minutes**

Exercise/Activity:

____

____

The Daily DASH Diet
2000 Calorie Plan (reduce or add food as needed)
Sodium Goal: 2300 mg/day or 1500 mg/day

Grains – 4-6 servings per day; try for whole grains
☐ ☐ ☐ ☐ ☐ ☐

Vegetables – 4-6 servings per day; (serving = ½ c)
☐ ☐ ☐ ☐ ☐ ☐

Fruit – 4-6 servings per day; (serving= ½ c.)
☐ ☐ ☐ ☐ ☐ ☐

Milk & Milk Products – 2-3 servings (serving = 8 oz)
☐ ☐ ☐

Meat, Chicken, Fish – 6 servings (1 serving =1oz)
☐ ☐ ☐ ☐ ☐ ☐

Nuts, seeds, and legumes -- 4–5 per week
☐ ☐ ☐ ☐ ☐ ☐

Fats and oils – 2-3 per day
☐ ☐ ☐

Sweets and sugar – 5 servings or less per week
☐ ☐ ☐ ☐ ☐

How did you do today? √

A great day ☐ **Mostly followed DASH**☐ **I'll do better tomorrow** ☐

Your thoughts and feelings about dieting so far:

____

____

____

DAY 48 Date: ___________

Time	Food	Comments

6-8 8 oz. glasses of water √ ☐ ☐ ☐ ☐ ☐ ☐ ☐ ☐

Exercise? ☐ **Yes** ☐ **No** __________ **minutes**

Exercise/Activity:

____

____

The Daily DASH Diet
2000 Calorie Plan (reduce or add food as needed)
Sodium Goal: 2300 mg/day or 1500 mg/day

Grains – 4-6 servings per day; try for whole grains
☐ ☐ ☐ ☐ ☐ ☐

Vegetables – 4-6 servings per day; (serving = ½ c)
☐ ☐ ☐ ☐ ☐ ☐

Fruit – 4-6 servings per day; (serving= ½ c.)
☐ ☐ ☐ ☐ ☐ ☐

Milk & Milk Products – 2-3 servings (serving = 8 oz)
☐ ☐ ☐

Meat, Chicken, Fish – 6 servings (1 serving =1oz)
☐ ☐ ☐ ☐ ☐ ☐

Nuts, seeds, and legumes -- 4–5 per week
☐ ☐ ☐ ☐ ☐ ☐

Fats and oils – 2-3 per day
☐ ☐ ☐

Sweets and sugar – 5 servings or less per week
☐ ☐ ☐ ☐ ☐

How did you do today? √

A great day ☐ **Mostly followed DASH**☐ **I'll do better tomorrow** ☐

Your thoughts and feelings about dieting so far:

____

____

____

DAY 49 **Date: ____________**

Time	Food	Comments

6-8 8 oz. glasses of water √ ☐ ☐ ☐ ☐ ☐ ☐ ☐ ☐

Exercise? ☐ **Yes** ☐ **No** _________ **minutes**

Exercise/Activity:

____

____

The Daily DASH Diet
2000 Calorie Plan (reduce or add food as needed)
Sodium Goal: 2300 mg/day or 1500 mg/day

Grains – 4-6 servings per day; try for whole grains
☐ ☐ ☐ ☐ ☐ ☐

Vegetables – 4-6 servings per day; (serving = ½ c)
☐ ☐ ☐ ☐ ☐ ☐

Fruit – 4-6 servings per day; (serving= ½ c.)
☐ ☐ ☐ ☐ ☐ ☐

Milk & Milk Products – 2-3 servings (serving = 8 oz)
☐ ☐ ☐

Meat, Chicken, Fish – 6 servings (1 serving =1oz)
☐ ☐ ☐ ☐ ☐ ☐

Nuts, seeds, and legumes -- 4–5 per week
☐ ☐ ☐ ☐ ☐ ☐

Fats and oils – 2-3 per day
☐ ☐ ☐

Sweets and sugar – 5 servings or less per week
☐ ☐ ☐ ☐ ☐

How did you do today? √

A great day ☐ **Mostly followed DASH**☐ **I'll do better tomorrow** ☐

Your thoughts and feelings about dieting so far:

____

____

____

DAY 50

Date: ___________

Time	Food	Comments

6-8 8 oz. glasses of water √ ☐ ☐ ☐ ☐ ☐ ☐ ☐ ☐

Exercise? ☐ **Yes** ☐ **No** _________ **minutes**

Exercise/Activity:

____

____

The Daily DASH Diet
2000 Calorie Plan (reduce or add food as needed)
Sodium Goal: 2300 mg/day or 1500 mg/day

Grains – 4-6 servings per day; try for whole grains
☐ ☐ ☐ ☐ ☐ ☐

Vegetables – 4-6 servings per day; (serving = ½ c)
☐ ☐ ☐ ☐ ☐ ☐

Fruit – 4-6 servings per day; (serving= ½ c.)
☐ ☐ ☐ ☐ ☐ ☐

Milk & Milk Products – 2-3 servings (serving = 8 oz)
☐ ☐ ☐

Meat, Chicken, Fish – 6 servings (1 serving =1oz)
☐ ☐ ☐ ☐ ☐ ☐

Nuts, seeds, and legumes -- 4–5 per week
☐ ☐ ☐ ☐ ☐ ☐

Fats and oils – 2-3 per day
☐ ☐ ☐

Sweets and sugar – 5 servings or less per week
☐ ☐ ☐ ☐ ☐

How did you do today? √

A great day ☐ **Mostly followed DASH**☐ **I'll do better tomorrow** ☐

Your thoughts and feelings about dieting so far:

____

____

____

DAY 51 Date: ____________

Time	Food	Comments

6-8 8 oz. glasses of water √ ☐ ☐ ☐ ☐ ☐ ☐ ☐ ☐

Exercise? ☐ **Yes** ☐ **No** _________ **minutes**

Exercise/Activity:

____

____

The Daily DASH Diet
2000 Calorie Plan (reduce or add food as needed)
Sodium Goal: 2300 mg/day or 1500 mg/day

Grains – 4-6 servings per day; try for whole grains
☐ ☐ ☐ ☐ ☐ ☐

Vegetables – 4-6 servings per day; (serving = ½ c)
☐ ☐ ☐ ☐ ☐ ☐

Fruit – 4-6 servings per day; (serving= ½ c.)
☐ ☐ ☐ ☐ ☐ ☐

Milk & Milk Products – 2-3 servings (serving = 8 oz)
☐ ☐ ☐

Meat, Chicken, Fish – 6 servings (1 serving =1oz)
☐ ☐ ☐ ☐ ☐ ☐

Nuts, seeds, and legumes -- 4–5 per week
☐ ☐ ☐ ☐ ☐ ☐

Fats and oils – 2-3 per day
☐ ☐ ☐

Sweets and sugar – 5 servings or less per week
☐ ☐ ☐ ☐ ☐

How did you do today? √

A great day ☐ **Mostly followed DASH**☐ **I'll do better tomorrow** ☐

Your thoughts and feelings about dieting so far:

____

____

____

DAY **52** Date: ____________

Time	Food	Comments

6-8 8 oz. glasses of water √ ☐ ☐ ☐ ☐ ☐ ☐ ☐ ☐

Exercise? ☐ **Yes** ☐ **No** ________ **minutes**

Exercise/Activity:

____

____

The Daily DASH Diet
2000 Calorie Plan (reduce or add food as needed)
Sodium Goal: 2300 mg/day or 1500 mg/day

Grains – 4-6 servings per day; try for whole grains
☐ ☐ ☐ ☐ ☐ ☐

Vegetables – 4-6 servings per day; (serving = ½ c)
☐ ☐ ☐ ☐ ☐ ☐

Fruit – 4-6 servings per day; (serving= ½ c.)
☐ ☐ ☐ ☐ ☐ ☐

Milk & Milk Products – 2-3 servings (serving = 8 oz)
☐ ☐ ☐

Meat, Chicken, Fish – 6 servings (1 serving =1oz)
☐ ☐ ☐ ☐ ☐ ☐

Nuts, seeds, and legumes -- 4–5 per week
☐ ☐ ☐ ☐ ☐ ☐

Fats and oils – 2-3 per day
☐ ☐ ☐

Sweets and sugar – 5 servings or less per week
☐ ☐ ☐ ☐ ☐

How did you do today? √

A great day ☐ **Mostly followed DASH**☐ **I'll do better tomorrow** ☐

Your thoughts and feelings about dieting so far:

____

____

____

DAY **53** Date: ___________

Time	Food	Comments

6-8 8 oz. glasses of water √ ☐ ☐ ☐ ☐ ☐ ☐ ☐ ☐

Exercise? ☐ **Yes** ☐ **No** _________ **minutes**

Exercise/Activity:

____

____

The Daily DASH Diet
2000 Calorie Plan (reduce or add food as needed)
Sodium Goal: 2300 mg/day or 1500 mg/day

Grains – 4-6 servings per day; try for whole grains
☐ ☐ ☐ ☐ ☐ ☐

Vegetables – 4-6 servings per day; (serving = ½ c)
☐ ☐ ☐ ☐ ☐ ☐

Fruit – 4-6 servings per day; (serving= ½ c.)
☐ ☐ ☐ ☐ ☐ ☐

Milk & Milk Products – 2-3 servings (serving = 8 oz)
☐ ☐ ☐

Meat, Chicken, Fish – 6 servings (1 serving =1oz)
☐ ☐ ☐ ☐ ☐ ☐

Nuts, seeds, and legumes -- 4–5 per week
☐ ☐ ☐ ☐ ☐ ☐

Fats and oils – 2-3 per day
☐ ☐ ☐

Sweets and sugar – 5 servings or less per week
☐ ☐ ☐ ☐ ☐

How did you do today? √

A great day ☐ **Mostly followed DASH**☐ **I'll do better tomorrow** ☐

Your thoughts and feelings about dieting so far:

____

____

____

DAY **54**

Date: ____________

Time	Food	Comments

6-8 8 oz. glasses of water √ ☐ ☐ ☐ ☐ ☐ ☐ ☐ ☐

Exercise? ☐ **Yes** ☐ **No** _________ **minutes**

Exercise/Activity:

____

____

The Daily DASH Diet
2000 Calorie Plan (reduce or add food as needed)
Sodium Goal: 2300 mg/day or 1500 mg/day

Grains – 4-6 servings per day; try for whole grains
☐ ☐ ☐ ☐ ☐ ☐

Vegetables – 4-6 servings per day; (serving = ½ c)
☐ ☐ ☐ ☐ ☐ ☐

Fruit – 4-6 servings per day; (serving= ½ c.)
☐ ☐ ☐ ☐ ☐ ☐

Milk & Milk Products – 2-3 servings (serving = 8 oz)
☐ ☐ ☐

Meat, Chicken, Fish – 6 servings (1 serving =1oz)
☐ ☐ ☐ ☐ ☐ ☐

Nuts, seeds, and legumes -- 4–5 per week
☐ ☐ ☐ ☐ ☐ ☐

Fats and oils – 2-3 per day
☐ ☐ ☐

Sweets and sugar – 5 servings or less per week
☐ ☐ ☐ ☐ ☐

How did you do today? √

A great day ☐ **Mostly followed DASH**☐ **I'll do better tomorrow** ☐

Your thoughts and feelings about dieting so far:

____

____

____

DAY 55 Date: ___________

Time	Food	Comments

6-8 8 oz. glasses of water √ ☐ ☐ ☐ ☐ ☐ ☐ ☐ ☐

Exercise? ☐ **Yes** ☐ **No** _________ **minutes**

Exercise/Activity:

____

____

The Daily DASH Diet
2000 Calorie Plan (reduce or add food as needed)
Sodium Goal: 2300 mg/day or 1500 mg/day

Grains – 4-6 servings per day; try for whole grains
☐ ☐ ☐ ☐ ☐ ☐

Vegetables – 4-6 servings per day; (serving = ½ c)
☐ ☐ ☐ ☐ ☐ ☐

Fruit – 4-6 servings per day; (serving= ½ c.)
☐ ☐ ☐ ☐ ☐ ☐

Milk & Milk Products – 2-3 servings (serving = 8 oz)
☐ ☐ ☐

Meat, Chicken, Fish – 6 servings (1 serving =1oz)
☐ ☐ ☐ ☐ ☐ ☐

Nuts, seeds, and legumes -- 4–5 per week
☐ ☐ ☐ ☐ ☐ ☐

Fats and oils – 2-3 per day
☐ ☐ ☐

Sweets and sugar – 5 servings or less per week
☐ ☐ ☐ ☐ ☐

How did you do today? √

A great day ☐ **Mostly followed DASH**☐ **I'll do better tomorrow** ☐

Your thoughts and feelings about dieting so far:

____

____

____

DAY **56**

Date: ___________

Time	Food	Comments

6-8 8 oz. glasses of water √ ☐ ☐ ☐ ☐ ☐ ☐ ☐ ☐

Exercise? ☐ **Yes** ☐ **No** _________ **minutes**

Exercise/Activity:

____

____

The Daily DASH Diet

2000 Calorie Plan (reduce or add food as needed)

Sodium Goal: 2300 mg/day or 1500 mg/day

Grains – 4-6 servings per day; try for whole grains

☐ ☐ ☐ ☐ ☐ ☐

Vegetables – 4-6 servings per day; (serving = ½ c)

☐ ☐ ☐ ☐ ☐ ☐

Fruit – 4-6 servings per day; (serving= ½ c.)

☐ ☐ ☐ ☐ ☐ ☐

Milk & Milk Products – 2-3 servings (serving = 8 oz)

☐ ☐ ☐

Meat, Chicken, Fish – 6 servings (1 serving =1oz)

☐ ☐ ☐ ☐ ☐ ☐

Nuts, seeds, and legumes -- 4–5 per week

☐ ☐ ☐ ☐ ☐ ☐

Fats and oils – 2-3 per day

☐ ☐ ☐

Sweets and sugar – 5 servings or less per week

☐ ☐ ☐ ☐ ☐

How did you do today? √

A great day ☐ **Mostly followed DASH**☐ **I'll do better tomorrow** ☐

Your thoughts and feelings about dieting so far:

____

____

____

DAY 57 Date: ____________

Time	Food	Comments

6-8 8 oz. glasses of water √ ☐ ☐ ☐ ☐ ☐ ☐ ☐ ☐

Exercise? ☐ **Yes** ☐ **No** ________ **minutes**

Exercise/Activity:

____

____

The Daily DASH Diet
2000 Calorie Plan (reduce or add food as needed)
Sodium Goal: 2300 mg/day or 1500 mg/day

Grains – 4-6 servings per day; try for whole grains
☐ ☐ ☐ ☐ ☐ ☐

Vegetables – 4-6 servings per day; (serving = ½ c)
☐ ☐ ☐ ☐ ☐ ☐

Fruit – 4-6 servings per day; (serving= ½ c.)
☐ ☐ ☐ ☐ ☐ ☐

Milk & Milk Products – 2-3 servings (serving = 8 oz)
☐ ☐ ☐

Meat, Chicken, Fish – 6 servings (1 serving =1oz)
☐ ☐ ☐ ☐ ☐ ☐

Nuts, seeds, and legumes -- 4–5 per week
☐ ☐ ☐ ☐ ☐ ☐

Fats and oils – 2-3 per day
☐ ☐ ☐

Sweets and sugar – 5 servings or less per week
☐ ☐ ☐ ☐ ☐

How did you do today? √

A great day ☐ **Mostly followed DASH**☐ **I'll do better tomorrow** ☐

Your thoughts and feelings about dieting so far:

____

____

____

DAY 58

Date: ___________

Time	Food	Comments

6-8 8 oz. glasses of water √ ☐ ☐ ☐ ☐ ☐ ☐ ☐ ☐

Exercise? ☐ **Yes** ☐ **No** _________ **minutes**

Exercise/Activity:

____

____

The Daily DASH Diet
2000 Calorie Plan (reduce or add food as needed)
Sodium Goal: 2300 mg/day or 1500 mg/day

Grains – 4-6 servings per day; try for whole grains
☐ ☐ ☐ ☐ ☐ ☐

Vegetables – 4-6 servings per day; (serving = ½ c)
☐ ☐ ☐ ☐ ☐ ☐

Fruit – 4-6 servings per day; (serving= ½ c.)
☐ ☐ ☐ ☐ ☐ ☐

Milk & Milk Products – 2-3 servings (serving = 8 oz)
☐ ☐ ☐

Meat, Chicken, Fish – 6 servings (1 serving =1oz)
☐ ☐ ☐ ☐ ☐ ☐

Nuts, seeds, and legumes -- 4–5 per week
☐ ☐ ☐ ☐ ☐ ☐

Fats and oils – 2-3 per day
☐ ☐ ☐

Sweets and sugar – 5 servings or less per week
☐ ☐ ☐ ☐ ☐

How did you do today? √

A great day ☐ **Mostly followed DASH**☐ **I'll do better tomorrow** ☐

Your thoughts and feelings about dieting so far:

____

____

____

DAY 59 **Date: ____________**

Time	Food	Comments

6-8 8 oz. glasses of water √ ☐ ☐ ☐ ☐ ☐ ☐ ☐ ☐

Exercise? ☐ Yes ☐ No _________ minutes

Exercise/Activity:

____

____

The Daily DASH Diet
2000 Calorie Plan (reduce or add food as needed)
Sodium Goal: 2300 mg/day or 1500 mg/day

Grains – 4-6 servings per day; try for whole grains
☐ ☐ ☐ ☐ ☐ ☐

Vegetables – 4-6 servings per day; (serving = ½ c)
☐ ☐ ☐ ☐ ☐ ☐

Fruit – 4-6 servings per day; (serving= ½ c.)
☐ ☐ ☐ ☐ ☐ ☐

Milk & Milk Products – 2-3 servings (serving = 8 oz)
☐ ☐ ☐

Meat, Chicken, Fish – 6 servings (1 serving =1oz)
☐ ☐ ☐ ☐ ☐ ☐

Nuts, seeds, and legumes -- 4–5 per week
☐ ☐ ☐ ☐ ☐ ☐

Fats and oils – 2-3 per day
☐ ☐ ☐

Sweets and sugar – 5 servings or less per week
☐ ☐ ☐ ☐ ☐

How did you do today? √

A great day ☐ Mostly followed DASH☐ I'll do better tomorrow ☐

Your thoughts and feelings about dieting so far:

____

____

____

DAY 60

Date: ____________

Time	Food	Comments

6-8 8 oz. glasses of water √ ☐ ☐ ☐ ☐ ☐ ☐ ☐ ☐

Exercise? ☐ **Yes** ☐ **No** _________ **minutes**

Exercise/Activity:

____

____

The Daily DASH Diet
2000 Calorie Plan (reduce or add food as needed)
Sodium Goal: 2300 mg/day or 1500 mg/day

Grains – 4-6 servings per day; try for whole grains
☐ ☐ ☐ ☐ ☐ ☐
Vegetables – 4-6 servings per day; (serving = ½ c)
☐ ☐ ☐ ☐ ☐ ☐
Fruit – 4-6 servings per day; (serving= ½ c.)
☐ ☐ ☐ ☐ ☐ ☐
Milk & Milk Products – 2-3 servings (serving = 8 oz)
☐ ☐ ☐
Meat, Chicken, Fish – 6 servings (1 serving =1oz)
☐ ☐ ☐ ☐ ☐ ☐
Nuts, seeds, and legumes -- 4–5 per week
☐ ☐ ☐ ☐ ☐ ☐
Fats and oils – 2-3 per day
☐ ☐ ☐
Sweets and sugar – 5 servings or less per week
☐ ☐ ☐ ☐ ☐

How did you do today? √

A great day ☐ **Mostly followed DASH**☐ **I'll do better tomorrow** ☐

Your thoughts and feelings about dieting so far:

____

____

____

DAY Date: ____________

Time	Food	Comments

6-8 8 oz. glasses of water √ ☐ ☐ ☐ ☐ ☐ ☐ ☐ ☐

Exercise? ☐ **Yes** ☐ **No** _________ **minutes**

Exercise/Activity:

____

____

The Daily DASH Diet
2000 Calorie Plan (reduce or add food as needed)
Sodium Goal: 2300 mg/day or 1500 mg/day

Grains – 4-6 servings per day; try for whole grains
☐ ☐ ☐ ☐ ☐ ☐

Vegetables – 4-6 servings per day; (serving = ½ c)
☐ ☐ ☐ ☐ ☐ ☐

Fruit – 4-6 servings per day; (serving= ½ c.)
☐ ☐ ☐ ☐ ☐ ☐

Milk & Milk Products – 2-3 servings (serving = 8 oz)
☐ ☐ ☐

Meat, Chicken, Fish – 6 servings (1 serving =1oz)
☐ ☐ ☐ ☐ ☐ ☐

Nuts, seeds, and legumes -- 4–5 per week
☐ ☐ ☐ ☐ ☐ ☐

Fats and oils – 2-3 per day
☐ ☐ ☐

Sweets and sugar – 5 servings or less per week
☐ ☐ ☐ ☐ ☐

How did you do today? √

A great day ☐ **Mostly followed DASH**☐ **I'll do better tomorrow** ☐

Your thoughts and feelings about dieting so far:

____

____

____

DAY

Date: ____________

Time	Food	Comments

6-8 8 oz. glasses of water √ ☐ ☐ ☐ ☐ ☐ ☐ ☐ ☐

Exercise? ☐ **Yes** ☐ **No** _________ **minutes**

Exercise/Activity:

____

____

The Daily DASH Diet
2000 Calorie Plan (reduce or add food as needed)
Sodium Goal: 2300 mg/day or 1500 mg/day

Grains – 4-6 servings per day; try for whole grains
☐ ☐ ☐ ☐ ☐ ☐

Vegetables – 4-6 servings per day; (serving = ½ c)
☐ ☐ ☐ ☐ ☐ ☐

Fruit – 4-6 servings per day; (serving= ½ c.)
☐ ☐ ☐ ☐ ☐ ☐

Milk & Milk Products – 2-3 servings (serving = 8 oz)
☐ ☐ ☐

Meat, Chicken, Fish – 6 servings (1 serving =1oz)
☐ ☐ ☐ ☐ ☐ ☐

Nuts, seeds, and legumes -- 4–5 per week
☐ ☐ ☐ ☐ ☐ ☐

Fats and oils – 2-3 per day
☐ ☐ ☐

Sweets and sugar – 5 servings or less per week
☐ ☐ ☐ ☐ ☐

How did you do today? √

A great day ☐ **Mostly followed DASH**☐ **I'll do better tomorrow** ☐

Your thoughts and feelings about dieting so far:

____

____

____

DAY **Date: ____________**

Time	Food	Comments

6-8 8 oz. glasses of water √ ☐ ☐ ☐ ☐ ☐ ☐ ☐ ☐

Exercise? ☐ **Yes** ☐ **No** _________ **minutes**

Exercise/Activity:

____

____

The Daily DASH Diet
2000 Calorie Plan (reduce or add food as needed)
Sodium Goal: 2300 mg/day or 1500 mg/day

Grains – 4-6 servings per day; try for whole grains
☐ ☐ ☐ ☐ ☐ ☐

Vegetables – 4-6 servings per day; (serving = ½ c)
☐ ☐ ☐ ☐ ☐ ☐

Fruit – 4-6 servings per day; (serving= ½ c.)
☐ ☐ ☐ ☐ ☐ ☐

Milk & Milk Products – 2-3 servings (serving = 8 oz)
☐ ☐ ☐

Meat, Chicken, Fish – 6 servings (1 serving =1oz)
☐ ☐ ☐ ☐ ☐ ☐

Nuts, seeds, and legumes -- 4–5 per week
☐ ☐ ☐ ☐ ☐ ☐

Fats and oils – 2-3 per day
☐ ☐ ☐

Sweets and sugar – 5 servings or less per week
☐ ☐ ☐ ☐ ☐

How did you do today? √

A great day ☐ **Mostly followed DASH**☐ **I'll do better tomorrow** ☐

Your thoughts and feelings about dieting so far:

____

____

____

References

Much of the content of this book originated in the writings and research from various agencies of the U.S. government, particularly NHLBI's "Your Guide to Lowering Your Blood Pressure with DASH", "Your Guide to Phiysical Activity and Your Heart" –NHLBI/DHHS. and the CDC's "Overweight and Obesity". Their websites, as well as other useful references, are noted below.

"Your Guide To Physical Activity and Your Heart"
U.S. Department of Health and Human Services
National Institutes of Health
National Heart, Lung, and Blood Institute
http://hp2010.nhlbihin.net/yourguide

"What Are the Health Risks of Overweight and Obesity?"
from the National Heart, Lung and Blood Institute (NIH).
http://www.nhlbi.nih.gov/health/health-topics/topics/obe/

NHLBI Health Information Center
Blood Pressure, Sodium and DASH—assorted resources
P.O. Box 30105
Bethesda, MD 20824-0105
Phone: 301-592-8573
TTY: 240-629-3255
Fax: 301-592-8563
www.nhlbi.nih.gov

"Your Guide to Lowering High Blood Pressure With DASH"
http://hp2010.nhlbihin.net/yourguide

"Overweight and Obesity"
Center for Disease Control and Prevention
http://www.cdc.gov/obesity/index.html

American Diabetes Association
The American Diabetes Association has interactive online tools to help you evaluate your lifestyle and your BMI:
http://www.diabetes.org/food-and-fitness/fitness/weight-loss/assess-your-lifestyle/your-current-health/

NIH, NHLBI Obesity Education Initiative. Clinical Guidelines on the Identification, Evaluation, and Treatment of Overweight and Obesity in Adults. Available online:
http://www.nhlbi.nih.gov/guidelines/obesity/ob_gdlns.pdf

Center for Disease Control and Prevention
The CDC has a Body Mass Index (BMI) and explains how it works.
http://www.cdc.gov/healthyweight/assessing/bmi/index.html

"Aim for a Healthy Weight"
A weightloss booklet from the NHLBI (National Heart, Lung and Blood Institute
http://www.nhlbi.nih.gov/health/public/heart/obesity/aim_hwt.htm

"Choose My Plate.gov"
The USDA home page, this site has the U.S. government's nutrition information and advice to encourage healthy eating habits.

"Dietary Guidelines for Americans 2010"
The Department of Health and Human Services (HHS) and the Department of Agriculture (USDA) publish this booklet of dietary and health advice together.

DHHS
www.healthfinder.gov

Health Topics AZ Index:
www.nhlbi.nih.gov/health/health-topics/

Dietary Guidelines for Americans 2005 and A Healthier You:
www.healthierus.gov/dietaryguidelines/

How to Understand and Use the Nutrition Facts Label:
www.cfsan.fda.gov/~dms/foodlab.html

MyPyramid and other nutrition information:
www.mypyramid.gov and www.nutrition.gov

The President's Council on Physical Fitness and Sports: www.fitness.gov

Aim for a Healthy Weight:
http://healthyweight.nhlbi.nih.gov.

Your Guide to Lowering High Blood Pressure:
www.nhlbi.nih.gov/hbp/index.html

Live Healthier, Live Longer (on lowering elevated blood cholesterol): www.nhlbi.nih.gov/chd

U.S. News and World Repor, "Best Diets", http://health.usnews.com/best-diet

We Can! (Ways to Enhance Children's Activity and Nutrition): http://wecan.nhlbi.nih.gov or call toll-free at 1–866–35WECAN

President's Council on Physical Fitness: www.fitness.gov

For more information on heart health, see MedlinePlus: www.medlineplus.gov

Made in the USA
Lexington, KY
04 December 2013